GREEN IMMUNITY BOOSTERS

BOTANICALS FOR IMMUNITY

Beating Colds, Influenza, and Other Germs with
Olive Leaf Extract, ARA-Larix, and Andrographis

James B

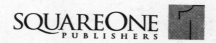

SQUAREONE
PUBLISHERS

Square One Publishers
115 Herricks Road
Garden City Park, NY 11040
516-535-2010 • 877-900-BOOK
www.squareonepublishers.com

ISBN 978-0-7570-0321-9

Copyright © 2009 by Square One Publishers

Printed in the United States of America

10 9 8 7 6 5 4 3 2 1

Contents

1

INTRODUCTION
BATTLEFIELD EARTH

Earth is a battlefield where bacteria and viruses have been at war with higher organisms for millions of years. Pathogenic bacteria and viruses view plants and animals—and yes, you and me—as large storehouses, filled with all the essential resources they need for survival. Indeed, we are the one-stop-shopping supermarket for pathogens. They will stop at nothing to steal our resources; they will hide, change appearance, test our defenses, and exploit our weaknesses. And if they fail the first time around, they will adapt and try again. Take SARS, for example.

In early 2003, a mysterious virus called Severe Acute Respiratory Syndrome (SARS) quickly spread to infect about 10,000 people across nearly 40 countries—but it was contained; proclaimed "eradicated" by the World Health Organization in 2004. While the lethality of SARS was below 1 percent for people under 25 years old, the prognosis was not so good for the rest of the population. Of the people who fell ill with the virus, it killed 6 percent of those aged 25 to 44, 15 percent of those 45 to 64, and more than 50 percent of those over 65.

In 2006, a different mysterious virus, called H5N1, or, more commonly, "bird flu," started to travel through bird populations the world over. Anxieties skyrocketed over bird flu's devastating pandemic potential—and justifiably so. Science has concluded that many flu strains that infect humans are actually mutated viruses that originated in other animals, such as pigs and chickens. Health organizations around the world fear that if bird flu (H5N1) mutates into a human-transmissible variant, the death toll will be catastrophic.

History gives us very sound reason to fear that a human variant will evolve. We need only look back at the 1918–1919 flu pandemic, known as the Spanish flu. This was arguably the worst influenza pandemic in history. It reached every corner of the globe, killing anywhere from 20 million to 100 million people in just two years. The genetic code of the Spanish flu, scientifically referred to as H1N1 virus, was recently found to be very closely related to that of the H5N1 bird flu virus of today. In fact, many researchers believe that Spanish flu started out as a bird flu virus before mutating into human-transmissible form (transmitted from one human to another). So, as we see bird populations, both domestic and wild, falling victim to H5N1, we can watch it evolve closer and closer to a human-transmissible form, which would likely become a super flu. In fact, as I write this, I see news reports of a variant having recently killed a woman in China. Further evolution may have allowed this variant to move swiftly to other people.

Meanwhile, the regular old seasonal flu wreaks havoc that is very real, and often overlooked. In fact, according to the National Institute of Allergy and Infectious Diseases, in the United States alone more than 100,000 people are hospitalized and more than 20,000 people die from the flu and its complications every year. Infants and the geriatric population are particularly at risk. The common cold adds another 100 million doctor's visits into the mix every year— and that's not including the countless millions who manage colds through home care alone. More frightening still, when the common cold has us down for the count, opportunistic infections such as bronchitis, strep throat, and pneumonia move in— exacerbating sickness from mere bedridden misery to a state of red-alert health danger.

Keep in mind, antibiotics are entirely ineffective against viruses. And even the latest antiviral drugs have proven ineffective against cold and flu viruses. Some reports suggest that 90% of flu viruses are resistant to Tamiflu, traditional medicine's supposed knight in shining armor. And the Associated Press reported in December 2008 that, "Early tests indicate that 49 of 50 samples of the main flu virus circulating this year—H1N1—were resistant to Tamiflu." To make matters worse, it took three years before initial concerns about psychiatric side effects were translated into formal label warnings announced in March 2008. According to newsinferno.com, "The FDA Tamiflu advisory panel had reviewed more than 600 cases of Tamiflu psychiatric side effects, including hallucinations and delirium. Many of those Tamiflu side effect reports involved children and some resulted in fatalities." If these reports are correct, this example of science's best weapon against influenza is not only an abysmal failure, but it also carries risks of frightening psychiatric side effects.

As these viruses shift, adapt, and make staggering biological leaps, scientists scramble to engineer new vaccines. But for the foreseeable future, an effective means of diffusing such pandemic time bombs as SARS, H5N1, and H1N1 remains beyond our capabilities. So most of us find ourselves doing little more than keeping our fingers crossed and hoping for the best. If you are reading this book, then you have decided to learn how to be more proactive about preventing and fighting back against cold and flu bugs. This book will teach you how three simple botanicals, readily available as dietary supplements at your local health food store, can help you to bolster your immune defenses.

Pharmaceutical companies get clearance to test only a handful of new vaccines, antibiotics, and antiviral drugs each year. In contrast, by the time we are about a year old, every human being has about a trillion different antibiotic and antiviral agents in our bones, ready and waiting to spring into battle to protect us. With a trillion different antibodies and immune cell warriors ever ready to battle our bacterial and viral enemies, it's a wonder that any foreign invader can penetrate our defenses and do us any harm at all.

Although preprogrammed to battle specific pathogens, very few humans have the resources needed to mount a timely and effective defense. It takes time for our immune systems to recognize a bacterium or virus and then sound the alarm. Then it takes even more time for the primordial immune cells to react, multiply, and ultimately send out the troops to stage a response. The primary reason bacteria and viruses are so successful against us is that they can often mount very quick surprise attacks, multiplying faster than our immune systems can counter.

This book will show you how to use safe and natural nutrients to heighten your immune cells' state of readiness. It will show you how to slow the proliferative progress of bacteria and viruses. And it will show you how to ensure that your immune system is prepared to respond as quickly as possible to any pathogenic threat.

2

UNDERSTANDING
THE ENEMY

In the Introduction, I mentioned that we are continually being attacked by bacteria and viruses, but many people have no idea what bacteria and viruses are. You can't see them. You can't smell them. But when your nose gets stuffy and you start coughing and feeling aches and pains, you sure know when they're around. But what exactly are they?

We know that the human body is composed of cells. Each cell is a living, breathing unit of life. Some can divide to form two cells. Some can continue to divide, creating millions of copies of themselves. But most cells of the adult human body cannot divide at all. Most of our cells are very specialized and carry out perhaps one or two primary functions; and that's all they do for an entire lifetime. In fact, most of our cells are so specialized that they cannot obtain the basic resources (food, water, oxygen) they need to sustain life. They depend on the trillions of other cells in the human body for their life-sustaining resources. Bacteria and viruses are similar to our cells in many ways, but different enough to be a problem.

BACTERIA

Bacteria are also composed of cells, much like those that make up our human tissues. But unlike our highly specialized cells, which cannot survive on their own, bacteria are like wild animals, fairly independent and capable of finding, attacking, and consuming their needed resources. But they don't attack the way a lioness attacks, where a hunter or group of hunters sees its prey and chases after it. Bacteria play a numbers game. When a bacterium successfully catches its prey, a human nose for example, it steals whatever resources it can grab before the human immune system can respond. While it is doing this, the bacterium divides into two—and then again, and over and over again, making billions of copies of itself. Each bacterium may also put out chemical irritants so that when their population is high enough and there is enough irritant being made, it causes the human nose to sneeze or the lungs to cough. With millions of bacteria carried away in the water vapor droplets of each sneeze or cough, and each sneeze or cough able to stay in the air for over four hours, the probability of one bacterium encountering another human nose is very high. This is particularly true in the winter, when human noses tend to congregate indoors. This example illustrates a bacterium that propagates through coughs and sneezes, but many other bacteria follow a similar pattern. Some bacteria are transmitted through other bodily fluids, like saliva or tear droplets, while others may be transmitted via the blood, in food, or even other, more creative and sneaky methods.

VIRUSES

Viruses are a bit more difficult to understand. They're not really alive and they're not really dead. Human cells and bacterial cells are clearly alive; they are fluid-filled sacks that contain all of the biological machinery, as well as the DNA programming, necessary to live, breathe, self-repair, sometimes multiply, and carry out their biological functions. Viruses don't carry any of this biological machinery. They are fragments of genetic material, usually DNA, which are capable of infiltrating a living cell and hijacking all of its biological machinery in order to create billions more copies of themselves. In so doing, the viruses usually destroy the cell they have infiltrated. Overproduction of many virus copies, as well as induced chemical changes, will cause the host cell(s) to burst, releasing the viruses into the cell's surroundings. When our bodies cough or sneeze, or sometimes simply exhale, these billions of virus copies then leave our bodies and go on to find new prey in much the same way bacteria do.

This method of attack and propagation, utilized by bacteria and viruses, brings up a good point on avoiding these diseases: Wash your hands frequently, after going to a restroom, and certainly before eating, drinking, handling food, or touching your eyes. The most common way to get the cold or flu is by breathing in the microscopic droplets of air sneezed or coughed out by an infected person. But you can also contract the flu (and many other viral as well as bacterial infections) simply by touching a surface like a countertop, a telephone, a keyboard, or a doorknob that was previously touched by someone infected with the flu.

What's the Difference Between the Cold and the Flu?

Influenza (flu) viruses and the common cold viruses are very different from one another, both genetically as well as in their appearance. The common cold, which is actually a group of similar viruses called rhinoviruses, are essentially fragments of DNA (deoxyribonucleic acid), the same as the genetic material that is in our chromosomes, which we pass on from generation to generation. Common cold rhinoviruses generally infect the upper respiratory tract: the nose, mouth, throat, and the large bronchi tubes of the lungs. The common cold causes chemical imbalances as well as the wholesale destruction of many of the cells in our airways. This causes our bodies to produce inflammation and results in symptoms such as low-grade fever, nasal congestion, and runny nose, as well as cough associated with the common cold.

The influenza virus, on the other hand, is made of a genetic material called RNA (ribonucleic acid), which is similar to our DNA, but different enough to make study and treatment of these pathogens a completely unique area of virology. These are referred to as retroviruses. To illustrate the difference: the common cold uses DNA (as do bacteria and humans) as its primary genetic material and RNA as an intermediate medium, a temporary copy of genetic instructions for producing the cell's machinery. But retroviruses, composed of RNA, start out as the intermediary information and then hijack the host cell's machinery (and often its DNA), to carry out its purposes.

Influenza often affects the same tissues as the common cold, but it also can affect the stomach and intestines. Typically, you will experience a higher fever, many more body aches and chills, and much more fatigue with the flu. If you also have gastrointestinal discomfort and/or diarrhea, then it is more likely to be a case of influenza rather than a common cold.

The reason I discuss the differences between the common cold and influenza viruses is not to help you self-diagnose, but rather, to give you an idea of the very different nature of these two pathogens. Researchers agree that there are approximately 200 to 300 different rhinovirus strains that we casually refer to as the common cold. They say that these strains have been infecting humans for millennia, and they are genetically relatively stable. That is, they don't mutate into new forms very quickly. So, if you have caught every one of the 200 to 300 different kinds of common cold viruses in existence, chances are that you will be immune. Your immune system has a pretty good memory and will be able to quickly conquer almost any cold virus it has seen before. This is good news, because it shows that, at least theoretically, a vaccine for the common cold—which would have to be a vaccine against 200 to 300 different rhinoviruses—could actually work. Of course, that essentially means making 300 individual vaccines and then combining them. Creating a vaccine would be a significant medical achievement, and is certainly many years off. And, of course, there is the problem of asking your immune system to respond to so many vaccines at once.

But the situation with influenza viruses is much different. Unlike the genetically stable common cold, the RNA-based influenza virus has a highly unstable set of genes within its genetic code. That area of instability governs the structure of the outer shell of the virus. Many viruses cause the host cell to create the viral outer shell material. Then, prior to rupturing the host cell, each virus will wrap itself in that shell material, so that when it goes out into the environment it has a protective shell, called a capsid, to shield against the elements. In the case of influenza, the genes responsible for that outer shell mutate frequently. As a result, the influenza virus that our bodies were able to identify and destroy last year may have mutated so much that by the time it comes around again during this cold and flu season, our immune systems no longer recognize it. The newly mutated flu viruses will now have the upper hand and catch our immune systems off guard. Flu vaccines have been deemed by the CDC to be relatively ineffective over the last several years. This is principally because it is a guessing game as to which influenza strain should be used to make the vaccine. Since our immune system is specific in building a response to a vaccine, if the wrong flu strain is picked, we are still vulnerable. As for vaccinating infants, small children, and teens, the *Journal of Pediatrics and Adolescent Health Care* could not report a defined benefit from recent vaccinations for the flu.

A sensible strategy is to work at building a stronger defense. By increasing the number and activity of immune defensive cells on the lookout for countless different pathogens, you can increase the odds of recognizing the new flu virus and neutralizing its advantage of the element of surprise.

To make matters worse, influenza viruses can swap genetic material and create new variants, just as easily as they change coatings. The fact that some influenza viruses can infect two or more different species of animals makes this characteristic particularly dangerous for us humans. Imagine that one influenza virus strain is highly lethal. But it is only capable of killing pigs and birds. That lethal virus can infect a bird that is already infected with a very mild, non-lethal strain of flu virus capable of infecting birds and humans. By swapping genes with the mild "bird and human flu," the lethal "pig and bird flu" virus can acquire the genes necessary to infect humans. If that virus were to be transmitted from a bird or pig to a human, it could result in a human pandemic of apocalyptic proportions.

While lethal, pandemic flu viruses only come around about once a century, the fact of the matter is that human-transmissible variants of influenza frequently result from gene-swapping in other species. And such gene-swapping may even occur within humans who have contracted two different strains of the flu. According to disease trackers, any place you find people living in close proximity to livestock or other animals, there is a tremendous increase in the risk of developing human variants of influenza. Southeast Asia happens to have a very high density of such human-animal cohabitation. So it is not surprising to learn that most new variants of influenza originate in impoverished Southeast Asian communities, where people essentially live with their livestock. So, even if researchers were able to develop an effective vaccine against the common cold viruses (all 300 of them), we would not likely see a vaccine for influenza anytime soon. The fact that there is neither a vaccine nor a cure in sight, and given that a lethal pandemic flu may be just one cold and flu season away, is plenty of reason to learn how to naturally amplify and enhance the effectiveness of your own immune defenses.

Addendum: *At the time of the printing of this book, new research published in the February 12, 2009, online version of the journal* Science *effectively outdated a concept described earlier in this section. If proven valid, the new research renders obsolete the previous belief that rhinovirus genomes are relatively stable. As it turns out, the genetic codes of cold viruses appear just as unstable and easily mutated as those of influenza viruses. Researchers have now mapped out the genetic sequences of 109 common colds and found that these rhinoviruses routinely mutate and swap segments of their genetic code. The broad implication is that an effective vaccine is virtually impossible. Even if scientists were able to create a vaccine against all known cold viruses today, it would not likely be effective in a few months' time. Odds are that at least some of the highly variable progeny of today's rhinovirus would not include the proteins against which any particular vaccine might be targeted. In fact, the study's authors conclude that an attempt to create a rhinovirus vaccine would be like trying to hit a moving target (Sequencing and Analyses of All Known Human Rhinovirus Genomes Reveals Structure and Evolution. Palmenberg AC, Spiro D, Kuzmickas R, Wang S, Djikeng A, Rathe JA, Fraser-Liggett CM, Liggett SB. (12 February 2009)* Science *[DOI: 10.1126/science.1165557]).*

Beyond the Cold and Flu

Even though this book focuses on cold and flu
viruses, the methods I teach and the botanical medicines I recommend to help optimize your immune
defenses go far beyond these pathogens. In fact,
they will help you defend against most other diseases of microbial origin. Larch arabinogalactan
(ARA-Larix), olive leaf extract, and *Andrographis
paniculata* extract can be used to heighten and hasten the body's immune response. I have used each
of these agents with great success in practice over
the past decade. They cannot be considered an
absolute shield against all viral pathogens, but they
can give your body a decisive advantage, shorten-
ing the duration and reducing the discomfort
caused by a host of common diseases. The following is a list of the most common infectious diseases
that can be inhibited by optimizing your defenses.

COMMON DISEASES AND INFECTIONS AND THEIR MICROBIAL CAUSES

Condition	Bacteria	Fungus	Virus
Athlete's foot		•	
Chickenpox			•
Common cold			•
Diarrheal disease	•		•
Flu			•
Genital herpes			•
Meningitis	•		•
Pneumonia	•	•	•
Sinusitis	•	•	
Skin diseases	•	•	•
Strep throat	•		
Tuberculosis	•		
Urinary tract infection	•		
Vaginal infections	•	•	
Viral hepatitis			•

Source: Understanding Microbes in Sickness and Health. U.S. Department of Health and Human Services, National Institute of Health. National Institute of Allergy and Infectious Diseases. NIH Publication No. 06-4914 January 2006.

3

KNOW YOUR OWN DEFENSES

The immune system is one of nature's most magnificent masterpieces; a complex network of vessels, cells, tissues, and organs. For example, the lymphatic system is the backbone of our immune system. It includes lymphatic vessels and lymph fluid as well as organs such as the spleen, thymus, and tonsils. A great deal of immune activity occurs in the gastrointestinal tract. The reasons for this will become clearer as I discuss probiotics later in this chapter.

The most familiar elements of "the immune system" are antibodies and white blood cells. This chapter addresses key activities of the immune system as a whole and the importance of antibodies and white blood cells in that system. This basic overview of the immune system will help you understand terms like "immune defenses" and what exactly it is that is doing all the defending. When we later describe specific activities of immune-boosting botanicals, you will understand what part of the immune system is getting boosted.

The job of the immune system is to detect threats to the body and mount a defense. When operating properly, the immune system appropriately responds only to microbial pathogens such as bacteria, viruses, fungi, and parasites, or to certain toxins. Optimally, the immune system responds only to true threats or signals of threat to our bodies, and not to benign chemicals that are supposed to be in the body. The two characters in the immune system most famous for achieving this are the white blood cell and the antibody.

White Blood Cells: Most people are aware that there is a group of immune system cells called white blood cells. You may also know that these white blood cells are produced in the marrow of most of our largest bones, such as the humerus (of the upper arm) and femur (of the upper leg). The picture we have of a white blood cell is that of an amoeba-like cell, capable of engulfing and digesting (thereby destroying) invading microbes.

Antibodies: You may also be familiar with another component of the immune system, called the antibody. The antibody is usually depicted as a "Y-shaped" structure that has very sticky arms. These sticky arms cause bacteria or viruses or even toxin molecules to clump together, thus immobilizing them so that they can be destroyed or digested by the amoeba-like white blood cells.

SPECIFICITY (FINE TUNING)

This basic understanding of white blood cells and antibodies is correct, but it is also tremendously simplified. If we view all white blood cells as essentially the same virus- or bacteria-munching,

PacMan-like creatures, we cannot possibly explain how the immune system truly functions. In fact, there are many different types of white blood cells and many different types of antibodies, each with a very specific assignment to protect us from harm. It is the division of labor among these different types of immune system characters that allows them to perform the miraculous job of identifying and eliminating only those molecules that don't belong in the body, and thereby removing the unwanted organisms of which they are a part.

This miraculous function of discriminating friend from foe truly is an astounding feat. To begin with, white blood cells and antibodies work on the molecular level. That is, they recognize and are specifically targeted to molecules, not whole organisms. If the target molecule happens to be attached to a pathogenic bacterial cell, then that pathogen will soon be white blood cell lunch, too. The immune system doesn't care what the foreign molecule is attached to if it senses a foreign molecule that doesn't belong in the body; it treats it as an enemy.

So when these defenders recognize a harmful bacterium or virus, they are really recognizing unique molecules on the surface of that bacterium or virus. You can think of it as a fingerprint that is identified. Just like every fingerprint is different, every invader has its own distinct "fingerprint." But here's where their job gets tricky. The number of molecules that exists in nature is, for all practical purposes, infinite. And there are tens of thousands of different molecules and unique configurations of molecules that do actually have a purpose within the human body. And for each benign or beneficial molecule that exists in nature, there is at least one that is potentially harmful. Yet, somehow, the human immune system is able to tell the difference between a surface protein on a human arterial cell and a very similar surface protein on a salmonella bacterium. The immune system is like a good police detective. By reading the "fingerprint" and ignoring our own surface protein, the immune system identifies and arrests the salmonella surface protein.

INFLAMMATION: THE GOOD, THE BAD, AND THE UGLY

When you injure yourself—say, you stub your toe, or you sprain your ankle—the body sends out inflammatory chemicals to *protect* you from further injury and begin healing. A little inflammation, in other words, is a good thing. But when inflammation occurs out of proportion to the injury or threat, or continues well past the time it is needed (such as chronic inflammation), the immune system needs to be reined in. Keeping the body's reactions within a healthy range is called "modulation": the immune system reacts appropriately; that is, it neither overreacts nor fails to adequately react.

When Good Immune Systems Go Bad

An overactive immune system can cause problems that range from annoying (such as mild food or seasonal allergies) to life-threatening (such as ana-phylactic shock and autoimmune diseases, e.g., lupus erythematosus).

Allergies: Most of this book has dealt with immune system cells of the bone marrow and white blood cells that circulate throughout the body. However, there is another class of immune system cells that embed themselves into various tissues in which there is a need for more pronounced and immediate immune response. These immune cells can be found in the lining of the eyes, nose, mouth, intestines, and airways, because these tissues are at greater risk of encountering pathogens. They are your first defense against invaders. When working properly, these immune cells respond to actual bacterial or viral threats by deploying chemical messengers (histamines and other mediators) to surrounding cells in an attempt to block the invasion. The blocking mechanism is what we experience as a runny nose, watery eyes, and inflammation. It is an outflow of fluids designed to carry the newly arriving bacteria or viruses out of the body. But in people who suffer from allergies, pollen, dust, and other non-threatening substances trigger the same blocking mechanism.

Anaphylactic Shock: If the immune system is not carefully tuned to discriminate friend from foe, the result could be disastrous. Anaphylactic shock (more commonly known as an extreme allergic reaction) is where one's immune system overreacts to the presence of an invader or a molecule that looks like an invader from the environment (usually from foods) and causes a massive release of histamines from white blood cells, potentially closing the airway of the lungs and shutting down breathing.

Autoimmune Disorders/Diseases: Today, one in twelve Americans suffers from an autoimmune disorder. In autoimmune disorders, the immune system can no longer identify the fingerprint of the body's own proteins as safe proteins that belong in your body. Instead of accurately identifying foreign invaders, your immune system begins to attack your own organs and tissues. Some types of auto-immune disease are debilitating and can lead to an early death. If you don't treat the condition, the body's own immune system slowly destroys the patient. If you treat the condition with potent phar-maceutical therapies which are targeted at quieting the immune system, the progression of the disease can be slowed down. But complications from the drug therapy can seriously affect quality of life or even do more damage to the immune system. Dietary changes, detoxification, hormone modula-tion, stress reduction, and natural therapies can all add value to managing the progression of autoim-mune disorders.

THE STICKY BUSINESS OF ANTIBODIES AND WHITE BLOOD CELLS

Antibodies are the key to understanding many dif-ferent aspects of the immune response. Once you understand how antibodies work, you will easily grasp how other parts of the immune system work. The way that antibodies seem to be the basis for other critical features of the immune system is an excellent example of how Mother Nature takes one successful technology and replicates it, with various modifications, for other purposes.

Antibodies

The secret to the immune system's success lies in the highly unique, sticky tips of those Y-shaped antibodies. Antibodies are microscopic structures akin to ultra-strong glue balls that will stick to virtually anything. Of course, Mother Nature is far more ingenious than to rely on simple sticky glue that cannot discriminate good molecules from bad. Your antibodies know better than to stick to substances made by your own cells, and they also avoid gumming up substances that are nutritionally valuable to your body.

But when bacteria or viruses attack your body, this sticky property of antibodies is extremely useful. When invading bacterial cells, for example, enter the body, they must be confined to one area where they can easily be found by white blood cells and destroyed shortly thereafter. Antibodies each have two sticky ends. One end will stick to one invading bacterial cell while the other end sticks to another bacterial cell, tethering the two bacteria together. Many thousands of such antibodies stuck to the surface of each bacterium will completely immobilize an entire colony. With trillions of antibodies floating around the body's fluids, it's easy to see how large colonies of bacteria can be stopped and killed very quickly.

Every antibody is composed of two relatively simple pairs of proteins. And no antibody could function if it were not for the disulfide cross-linking that holds its four proteins together. The diagram below is a schematic representation of the structure of typical antibodies.

Schematic Representation of Antibody Structure

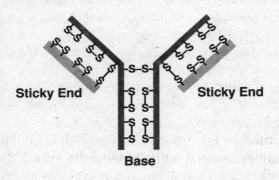

Each gray bar represents a protein, or chain of amino acids. With each "S" representing a sulfur atom, and each line connecting two sulfurs representing a disulfide bond, the diagram clearly shows the importance of sulfur in the structural integrity of antibodies. The reason there are so many disulfide bonds on such a small piece of protein is because the sticky ends must have an extremely precise structure. These sticky ends must allow a specific external molecule, and only that one specific molecule, to fit perfectly, like a lock and key within a groove formed by its unique structure. When the one and only molecule for which it was intended comes into contact with that sticky end, it falls into place like the key to a lock. And with such a good match, the antibody applies a very tight grip to the molecule. Hence that part of the antibody is often called "sticky."

You may be asking, "How does this one single antibody, which is only able to stick to one and only one molecule in the whole universe, translate to an immune system capable of discriminating among a trillion different friendly and unfriendly molecules?" If so, you're not alone; scientists took many years to answer this question on the most basic level. There are still many details that remain a mystery. But it all starts down in the bone marrow, and mostly takes place from about the time of birth until about a year later. This is where primordial white blood cells, which do not migrate from the bone marrow, happily divide, making many, many daughter cells. These daughter cells encode the genetic instructions on how to produce an antibody (millions of copies of that antibody). Each daughter cell is slightly different from the next, such that the genetic code would yield an antibody that recognizes—and sticks to—a slightly different molecule.

For about a year after birth, our bone marrow gets quickly populated with nearly a trillion such daughter cells, each ready to produce many copies of a single antibody which specifically binds a slightly different target molecule. This translates to about a trillion different molecular targets, and thus the potential to immobilize a trillion distinct microbes. By about one year of age, the human bone marrow is essentially ready to deploy antibodies against virtually any molecule Mother Nature can throw at it.

White Blood Cells

Recall how I said that understanding the antibody is the key to understanding the other characters of the immune system. Here's what I mean: The mechanism that enables those sticky ends of antibodies to recognize and bind one and only one molecule is the same mechanism that allows white blood cells to identify a specific molecule, and thereby the pathogen to which it is attached. Likewise, the mechanism that generates a trillion differently-targeted, antibody-producing cells is the same as that which generates a trillion differently-targeted white blood cells.

Each of these white blood cells recognizes friend or foe by using molecules on its surface that are very similar to antibodies. These are referred to as receptors. These receptors are so similar to antibodies that they are essentially modifications of antibodies, with most differences simply in structures that allow the base to anchor into the white blood cell. Also, while all antibodies have a "Y" shape, which consists of a base and two arms, receptors often have a base and only one arm. With the base firmly anchored into the white blood cell, the sticky ends (one or two) protrude into the cell's environment. When the white blood cell encounters a molecule to which the sticky end is targeted, it considers it a potential threat and goes into one of several modes, depending on what kind of white blood cell it is that has encountered the potential threat. Usually the response will either be "attack and destroy" or "sound the alarm": "Hey, everyone, I found an invader!"

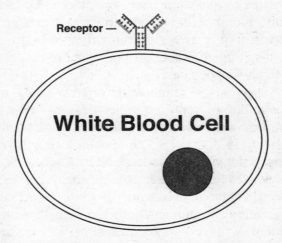

Some white blood cells simply patrol the circulatory system for molecules called "antigens." The term antigen describes a molecule, or even a part of a molecule, that produces a defensive response from the immune system. Optimally, our bodies would respond only to antigens that come from pathogenic organisms or toxins.

Once an antigen is found, the patrolling white blood cells initiate a chain of events that results in the presentation of the antigen to other white blood cells. These white blood cells confirm the threat, and in turn send signals to the previously described daughter cells, which are targeted to that one and only antigen molecule. While I've only described daughter cells that produce the amoeba-like white blood cells and antibody-producing cells, there are many other types of white blood cells that are targeted to that same specific antigen. All of these white blood cells respond to the alarm signal by performing many different functions to stop, destroy, and eliminate the pathogen from which the antigen was detected.

There are a number of steps involved in the recognition of pathogen molecules and in the communications between various cells of the immune system. In fact it is quite complex, with many aspects not yet fully understood by science. But it is known that if there are already many copies of a specific-pathogen-recognizing white blood cell in circulation throughout the body, then the immune system will recognize and attack that specific pathogen more quickly and easily than if there were fewer such immune cells floating around. Likewise, if there are more antibody-producing precursor cells ready and waiting, then the immune system will recognize and attack the specific pathogen far more quickly and easily than if there were fewer such cells ready and waiting in the bone marrow.

Vaccines

Actually, it is this readiness that modern vaccines hope to achieve. A vaccine is nothing more than an injection of unique proteins from a particular pathogen, which will cause your immune system to churn out millions and millions of white blood cells and antibodies specifically targeted to that pathogen. Then when you encounter a live bacterial or viral pathogen with the same target proteins, or fingerprint, your immune system will already have the antibodies and white blood cells programmed for a rapid response. There is a crucial balance between the value of vaccination and over-vaccination. A certain amount of immune challenge is necessary for the maturing of the immune system.

Beneficial Flora:
Digestion and Immune Health

A key factor in immune health is gastrointestinal health. This makes sense because practically every molecule in every cell, fluid, and tissue of your body got there via the gastrointestinal tract. (Wow! Stop and think about that: "You are what you eat" is very real.)

Consider that the digestive tract is the gateway through which many pathogens and toxins—as well as all beneficial nutrients from food—enter the body. With your immune system as gatekeeper, this is a very important place where "high fidelity" discrimination between friend and foe molecules must take place. So, while "you are what you eat" (or absorb), your immune system must make sure you are *not* what you *do not* absorb. When your immune cells recognize pathogens at their point of introduction to your body, you are in a better position to keep them from advancing. With trillions upon trillions of molecules transiting the gastrointestinal tract every minute of every day, the job of discriminating which are friendly and which are potentially harmful is simply incomprehensible. And the success achieved by the gastrointestinal tract in cooperation with the immune system in performing this function is nothing less than miraculous.

One of the most important factors that often affects the immune system's health is that of "probiotic balance." "Probiotics" refers to a number of bacteria that are actually beneficial and help us maintain good health. Probiotic balance is about keeping harmful intestinal bacteria in check. Improving probiotic balance alone can have a dramatic impact on the performance of your immune system. When combined with good immune-boosting botanicals, the effects can be even greater.

But in order to understand how probiotics work, we must understand some of the basics of the digestive tract. The process of digesting food relies on complex, interdependent chemical and enzymatic activities among the stomach, intestines, liver, pancreas, and so on. While all of the exact mechanisms of how friendly bacteria affect immune function are not fully understood, this much is true:

- Friendly bacteria (or microflora) in the intestines actually produce certain vitamins your body needs for healthy immune function (and other uses).

- Maintaining a healthy balance of intestinal microflora enables these complex, interdependent processes to operate as they should. You digest your food and your body receives nutrients for all of its structures and functions—including immune function. Good bacteria compete with bad bacteria for food; if the good bacteria's numbers are reduced, the bad bacteria can proliferate unchecked.

- When harmful intestinal bacteria get the upper hand, as can happen, for example, after a round of antibiotics or use of oral contraceptives, digestion is disrupted *and* the immune system is weakened. Alternatively, in a classic case of "the chicken or the egg": If digestion is compromised for whatever reason, the bad microflora can—and do—thrive. This can establish a vicious cycle of interfering with healthy digestion, robbing your body of the nutrition that sustains its activities, including immune function.

Just as the health of the digestive system depends on the health of the immune system, the reverse is also true: The health of the immune system depends on that of the digestive system. So, it is important to understand some of the factors that cause the digestive system to be healthy or unhealthy. Many tissues and organs—from the brain to the colon—are all involved in the proper functioning of the digestive system. But for our purposes, unfortunately we do not have the time to discuss roles of the mouth, throat, stomach, and brain-gut-immune communication, since our ultimate discussion is on the influence of probiotic bacteria, which reside in the intestines.

THE DETAILS OF DIGESTION

Remember from high school biology that hydrochloric acid in the stomach continues to break down the food that you have chewed and swallowed. What you may not have learned then (I don't think I did) is that stomach acid also kills many pathogens before passing partially-digested food down the line to the small intestine. (This initial destruction of pathogens is called "nonspecific immunity"; easy to remember because the specialized cells of the immune system are not yet involved. Naturally, the pH, or acidity, of the stomach strongly influences the degree to which it can destroy pathogens, in addition to breaking apart foods.) The fact that acid-blocking drugs are the number two category of prescription drugs tells you that there are many people needing immune support. This is because their first line of defense against pathogens is neutralized by the drug.

The small intestine—where partially digested food goes after leaving the stomach—is where most digestion actually occurs. It is critically important to remember that the small intestine is also where absorption of most nutrients into the bloodstream takes place. In fact, more than twelve major digestive enzymes and nearly all of the active mechanisms for nutrient absorption operate in the small intestine. The liver, the gallbladder, and the pancreas all play pivotal roles in the digestion and absorption of nutrients, because they release their digestive enzymes, fluids, and salts into the small intestine. Proper pH levels are needed for these digestive enzymes and salts, as well as for absorption of nutrients. The problem is, harmful intestinal bacteria can wreak havoc with pH, which results in changes in digestive and immune function.

Fat Digestion

You may remember from high school biology that the liver secretes bile, and that it is stored in the gallbladder until it is released into the first section of the small intestine (the duodenum) due to the presence of a meal. What you may not remember is that bile salts (or bile electrolytes, such as sodium and potassium) embedded in bile acid are the reason bile is so important to digestion. Such bile electrolytes allow for the breakdown of the fat droplets that enter the digestive tract as part of a meal. When fat enters the digestive tract, it is usually in the form of droplets of triglycerides, diglycerides, monoglycerides, and a small minority of free fatty acids. While these droplets may be microscopic on our scale, to a fat-digesting enzyme they are enormous, with the interior fat molecules entirely inaccessible. But in order to absorb that fat droplet, which often holds fat-soluble vitamins, such as A and D, and fat-soluble phytonutrients, such as beta-carotene, lutein, and lycopene, that fat droplet must be broken down into something more accessible to the fat-digesting enzymes, called lipase. Here's how its done.

Bile, which comes from the liver, is stored in the gallbladder until it is released into the first section of the small intestine (the duodenum) due to the presence of a meal. Bile acids and electrolytes, such as sodium and potassium, allow for the emulsification of dietary fats. This simply means that large fat globules are made into small droplets, miscible in the aqueous (watery) environs of the intestines. Making small droplets of dietary fats is important because lipase, fat-digesting enzymes, are water soluble and can only act on the fat molecules that happen to be on the outer surface of a fat droplet. Breaking up a large fat molecule into many smaller ones increases the surface area of fat molecules touching the watery environment. Lipase breaks triacylglycerols (triglycerides) and diacylglycerols (diglycerides) into monoacylglycerols (monoglycerides) and free fatty acids.

But bile's role is not yet over. Just as it facilitated the formation of smaller fat droplets, it also facilitates the formation of monoglycerides and free fatty acids into tiny spheres, called micelles. The cells lining the small intestine can easily absorb tiny micelles, and package their fatty acid molecules for transport in the blood.

Bile salts are so important to the digestion and absorption of fats that 94% of them are reabsorbed in the last part of the small intestine, called the ileum. (For anyone who may be misled by the notion that avoiding electrolytes may be a way of avoiding dietary fats for weight loss reasons, this is not recommended. Indeed, such a diet can be fatal, as electrolyte imbalance is a well-known cause of heart failure in otherwise healthy individuals.)

Carbohydrate and Protein Digestion and Further Digestion of Fats

The pancreas secretes a combination of substances, collectively known as pancreatic juice, into the duodenum. Pancreatic juice is just a little bit basic and has a pH of about 8.0. While the bile salts take care of most of the neutralization, the pancreatic juice is still partially responsible for the neutralization of the acid-soaked substances that have been passed from the stomach. Pancreatic juice also contains enzymes produced by the pancreas. These include carbohydrate-, protein-, and lipid-digesting enzymes, as well as RNA- and DNA-digesting enzymes. So we can see how our digestive system secretes digestive enzymes, and other agents such as bile salts, for virtually every kind of nutrient we are likely to encounter.

Now let's take a look at what can go wrong. Pancreatic secretions are stimulated primarily by the entrance of hydrochloric acid (HCl) from the stomach into the small intestine. (These secretions are also stimulated by the presence of the digested fragments and molecules of the foods we eat. However, both signals are necessary for a robust pancreatic response.) This tells you that HCl concentration and pH can have a tremendous influence enhancing or inhibiting one's ability to digest and absorb nutrients from the gastrointestinal tract into the bloodstream. In addition, the concentrations of specific enzymes can influence the digestion and subsequent absorption of a specific nutrient. (The concentrations of all of these substances are known to diminish as we get older). Yet, with the unavoidable presence of potentially harmful intestinal microorganisms, a lack of a particular enzyme or bile carries far more damaging consequences than an inability to assimilate a particular nutrient. If a person's digestive tract is unable to digest and absorb a nutrient, there are many harmful microorganisms that would be delighted to do so.

Such harmful microorganisms often also produce toxic or irritating substances called endotoxins, which can reduce HCl secretion in the stomach as well as secretions from the pancreas, liver, and gallbladder. If these harmful microorganisms can successfully colonize and thrive in your gastrointestinal tract, then the toxins they produce will reduce your ability to digest foods. Your inability to digest and absorb foods is exactly what the harmful bacteria want to happen, because if you cannot digest and absorb foods efficiently, then the unfriendly bacteria that live within you will have more unabsorbed food available for themselves. Harmful intestinal bacteria love to establish such vicious cycles; they cause improper digestion, which improves their ability to thrive, which causes more improper digestion, which further improves their ability to thrive. Unfortunately, such imbalances in the populations of harmful microorganisms can seriously diminish your immune response by:

- generally interfering with the recognition of pathogens from ingested substances,

- producing endotoxins that alter hormone, neurotransmitter, and immune signaling,

- reducing the nonspecific immunity of the stomach by inhibiting its HCl production, and

- reducing the vital nutrients your immune system needs in order to build defensive cells and structures.

So how do we regain control and balance in our gastrointestinal tract?

One important step is introducing probiotics, friendly intestinal microorganisms that have no adverse effects on human physiology. With colonies of probiotics firmly established in the gut, the nutrient resources available to the harmful intestinal bacteria are diminished. Thus, benign bacteria keep the populations of harmful bacteria in check. Probiotics are one of the most significant natural products that you can choose to use for regaining healthy immune function.

These probiotics are often referred to by their genus and species names, such as *Lactobacillus acidophilus, Lactobacillus bulgaricus, Lactobacillus sporogenes, Streptococcus thermophilus, Lactobacillus bifidus* (which was recently given its own genus, Bifidobacterium [*Bifidobacterium bifidus*]), and many others.

In addition to keeping bad bacteria in check, these probiotics naturally produce a number of vitamins and other nutrients useful to the human body. Most notably, they produce the B complex vitamins B1, B2, B12, biotin, folic acid, and pantothenic acid. And if these nutritional gifts were not enough, probiotic bacteria are also responsible for making many of the fermented foods that have kept many cultures deliciously fed for millennia. These include such foods as pickles; the fermented bean foods tempeh, miso, and doenjang; and yogurt and related foods such as kefir, kimchi, sauerkraut, and soy sauce.

For the purposes of this book, it is the range of benefits to our immune systems that is the most important activity of probiotics. Sufficient probiotic colonization and proper probiotic balance have been shown in numerous studies to improve a wide range of immune system activities. While most studies on the immune-enhancing effects have investigated the immune response as it pertains to the gastrointestinal tract, new research is showing benefits throughout the body.

One researcher, Dr. Karen Madsen of the University of Alberta, Division of Gastroenterology, recently published a review of the expanding role of probiotics in the treatment of critically ill patients suffering from a number of disorders, most of which are life-threatening. The benefits she notes are largely a result of improved immune function. And while her review stops shy of an outright recommendation, it does call attention to the growing importance of probiotics as adjunct therapy with many applications. (Madsen K. Probiotics in critically ill patients. *J Clin Gastroenterol.* 2008 Sep;42 Suppl 3 Pt 1:S116-8.).

As you will see later in this book, and particularly in the chapter on arabinogalactan, there is much you can do to improve the viability of probiotic bacteria while hindering that of harmful intestinal microbes.

WHAT DO WE MEAN BY "IMMUNE BOOSTING" ANYWAY?

We've talked about the specificity of individual immune system cells to identify countless unique microbial pathogens and other threats. We've also discussed the ability of certain cells to reproduce, on demand, millions of cells that will go forth and deal with the invaders. But due to factors that we address below, such as poor diet, stress, environmental pollution, and drug therapies (even when used appropriately), the ability of these cells to carry out their functions can be compromised; the immune system is effectively weakened. In this situation, for example, the white blood cells responsible for identifying invaders may not do so correctly or at all, take longer to do it, or may be too few in number to do the job. The cells that produce the millions of copies may be slow to act or may not produce enough cells to go after the replicating viral or bacterial cells. This is when the immune system needs a "boost," with "immune-enhancing" nutrients such as the phytochemicals in the natural botanicals we cover in this book.

Perhaps more than any other body system, it is our immune system that permits our bodies to be in a state of peak health and experience exhilarating well-being. When it's running like a fine-tuned machine, responding with appropriate force at the right time, the immune system is the most powerful defense we have against everything from the common cold to cancer. You can help support proper immune function through simple, natural changes in lifestyle and nutrition—including defense-bolstering botanicals like olive leaf, arabinogalactan, and andrographis. With the help of these supplements, you can strengthen a weakened immune system, modulate an overreacting immune system, and ensure that your natural internal defenses do their job in promoting peak health, vitality, and longevity.

4

YOUR IMMUNE SYSTEM VERSUS THE MODERN LIFESTYLE

All in all, as we have seen, there are many immune cell characters, each relying on good health and good working conditions. Many immune cells need optimal cellular health conditions to generate receptors with the exact, perfect shape needed to detect pathogen molecules and distinguish them from the myriad molecules that belong in the body. They must signal other immune cells. They must follow the instructions of yet other immune cells. They must travel through body tissues, lymphatic ducts, blood vessels, and other areas of the body to get to the scene of a bacterial or viral invasion. And then they must be ready to fight these germs.

Unfortunately, modern lifestyles and technology tend to make optimal immune health difficult to maintain. Furthermore, our modern environment tends to favor the propagation of pathogenic microorganisms.

While modern medicine fails to solve our most threatening health problems, the real frontline battle is fought entirely by our immune systems. Our

modern world has introduced factors that appear to
cripple nature's masterful immune system—leaving
our bodies weakened and susceptible to invading
pathogens. Here are six modern-day factors that
affect the immune system:

1. Overuse (and even use) of antibiotics
   and other drugs.
2. Poor nutritional status.
3. Modern agricultural practices.
4. Environmental and indoor pollution.
5. Overcrowding.
6. Chronic heightened stress.

Knowing these six factors as contributors to poor
immune function is vital to pre-empting or counter-
acting their effects.

Overuse of Antibiotics and Other Drugs

Antibiotics may be the wonder drugs of the 20th
Century, but they tend to rob the body of nutrients
and beneficial flora that are essential for optimal
immune health. Of course, when faced with the dil-
emma of mildly depressing a patient's immune system versus the potential damage that pathogenic bacteria can cause, most clinicians and patients will opt
in favor of the antibiotic treatment. But overuse of
antibiotics depresses our immunity far more than is
necessary. And, very few clinicians or patients follow
up a round of antibiotics with the appropriate measures to restore lost nutrients and probiotic balance.

By "overuse," I am referring to the following common scenarios:

1. If the doctor does not know what's bothering you, he may prescribe an antibiotic just in case the source of the illness is bacterial.

   Often, we have a common cold or flu, which are viral in nature and not affected by antibiotics. Yet we may feel pressure in our sinuses due to inflammation caused by our own immune response. Or we may feel gastrointestinal pain and nausea because it is a gastrointestinally active influenza virus. Or we may feel any number of symptoms that may lead us or our doctors to believe that the invading germ is different from the common cold or flu.

2. If the doctor does not prescribe *some*thing, anything, you may perceive that the doctor has done nothing to address your illness.

   When you are feeling miserable, it is disheartening to hear your healthcare practitioner tell you that there is nothing he or she can prescribe—the virus must simply run its course.

   Numerous investigations have found that physicians often prescribe antibiotics even though they know the drug will do nothing to shorten or ease the discomfort their patients are feeling. And many times parents pressure doctors into prescribing antibiotics. Doctors know that if they prescribe something, even unnecessarily, the patient feels as though he or she has been helped, and will feel more satisfied with the doctor's efforts. Fail to prescribe—even if to not prescribe anything is the best course of action—and many patients will feel that their doctor is not providing satisfactory service. This, of course, increases the risk of losing the patient to another physician who is all too eager to write unnecessary prescriptions.

Antibiotic-Resistant Super Germs

The most troublesome consequence of these prescribing habits is that the misuse of antibiotics is contributing to the rise of "super germs" that are resistant to antibiotics. Inappropriately prescribed antibiotics are no more likely to produce antibiotic-resistant germs than those that are appropriately prescribed. But, because each prescription carries the risk of contributing to the generation of an antibiotic-resistant strain, inappropriately prescribed antibiotics are an unnecessary risk.

The problem is that, with any antibiotic prescription, there is a risk that a few of the billions of bacteria it is intended to destroy will actually survive. Those that do survive have some tiny genetic difference that makes them just a little more capable of withstanding the antibiotic treatment than their billions of sibling germs were. Most likely, just a little more antibiotic treatment would have killed them. But in the end they survived. The offspring of that bacterium will all be slightly better capable of surviving such an antibiotic treatment than most bacteria of that species. The next person who gets infected by this line of bacteria may need a slightly stronger dose or have to take the antibiotics for slightly longer than the first person did in order to kill them all off. If a few bacteria survive this next round of antibiotics in the second person, then these will be even more capable of withstanding the antibiotic. After several generations, it is clear that the line of bacteria may become entirely unaffected by the antibiotic. Thus a "super germ" is born.

One of the worst things a patient can do—which will ensure that some bacteria survive toward the generation of such an antibiotic-resistant strain—is to not finish taking prescription antibiotics as directed. (How often have you or a family member done this?) Failing to complete a round of antibiotics ensures that a small number of bacteria will survive. If you do this, you are playing a significant part in the generation of an antibiotic-resistant strain of the very bacteria you are battling.

Some people start feeling better very quickly after starting antibiotics. Often this is a consequence of one's immune system naturally overcoming the germ. So they hold on to half the prescription and store it in their medicine cabinet in case they themselves or another family member comes down with the bug (or some other infection). The problem with this logic is that by the time the next family member comes down with a bacterial infection, the strain he or she comes down with may be resistant to the antibiotic, or there will not be a full prescription to use—not to mention that the prescription was intended only for one person. The misuse of antibiotics goes on every day, creating these super bugs. These sophisticated super bugs mutate in order to stay one step ahead of our best antibiotics. Meanwhile, we get sicker and the pathogens themselves get stronger [Sarker, P., & Gould, I. M. (2006). Antimicrobial agents are societal drugs. *Drugs*, 66(7), 893-901.]. This also forces the invention of more powerful antibiotics, which generally have more significant side effects.

One final note while we're on the subject of antibiotics. There is an increasing awareness from both clinicians and patients that antibiotics, even when prescribed appropriately, can rob the body of vital nutrients and the probiotic organisms needed for gastrointestinal health. But, doctors still rarely recommend taking probiotics during and after a round of antibiotics or with chronic maintenance. Even though it is prescribed with the intention of killing pathogenic bacteria, there's nothing stopping antibiotics from killing off the beneficial bacteria in your GI tract. In fact, that's exactly what happens most of the time. The

Considerations section of this book describes how to replenish your vitamins, minerals, and probiotics after a round of antibiotics.

Poor Nutritional Status

Americans are eating the worst diet in our history [Schuman, A. J. (2008). An obesity action plan. *Contemporary Pediatrics*, 25(4), 37-38, 41-42, 45-46.]. Many foods are not only deficient in the nutrition that is so crucial to peak immune function, but may also be loaded with sugar, preservatives, refined carbohydrates, and processed ingredients that can strengthen pathogens, weaken the immune defenses, and have a pro-inflammatory impact on the entire body, not limited to the sites of infection. Such needless, rampant inflammation can throw off the body's immune system even further, and potentially promote autoimmune diseases. What's worse, chronic inflammatory chemistry can increase the risk or progression of conditions and diseases that were previously considered unrelated to infection or inflammation. These include obesity, arthritis, heart disease, atherosclerosis, diabetes, and a host of other inflammation-related conditions.

Modern Agricultural Practices

Modern agricultural practices have also contributed to our declining immune function. Nutrient-deficient soil supplies less nutritious produce and may also increase the amount of pathogens in our environment. Viruses and bacteria thrive due to poor soil, surrounding us with potential illness [Marsh, D. E. (2006). Soil mineral deficiency and viral mutation: Nutritional, agricultural and geographic influences. *Positive Health*, 124, 28-31.]. Pesticides and herbicides also are routinely used to guarantee yield, with inadequate testing for safety and known immune-disrupting activity.

Additionally, antibiotics are used widely in ranching to prevent disease and increase yield, although studies have shown that 80% of these veterinary prophylactic antibiotic treatments are unnecessary and negatively impact our health and immune function. Dr. Eric Hentges, executive director of the U.S. Department of Agriculture's Center for Nutrition Policy and Promotion, has indicated a need for vitamins, minerals, and phytonutrients to be added to American diets to promote optimum health [Hentges, E. (2007). Promoting health with dietary guidance and My Pyramid: an interview with Eric Hentges, PhD. *Food Insight*, 1, 4-5.].

A last important aspect to agriculture is the fact that foods that have been modified for yield could have higher lectin content (type of protein) than traditional foods. This can make them more prone to becoming an allergenic food. Today's wheat, for example, has 40% more lectins than wheat of 50 years ago.

Environmental and Indoor Pollution

Environmental pollution overloads the immune system, potentially impairing its ability to ward off pathogens. These days, our bodies are constantly bombarded with microscopic toxic particles. Whether inhaled, ingested, or absorbed through the skin, these particles end up inside our bodies, where they're often detected as a threat by the immune system. Immune cells rush to dispose of these particles, but the toxic load places considerable stress on our defenses.

In addition to synthetic toxins, poor environmental conditions can breed incredible numbers of bacteria, which themselves may produce formidable toxins. For example, in Texas, researchers discovered that people living near animal storage or feeding lots were exposed to higher concentrations of antibiotic-resistant organisms than normal [Gibbs, S. G., Green, C. F., Tarwater, P. M., Mota, L. C., Mena, K. D., & Scarpino, P. V. (2006). Isolation of antibiotic-resistant bacteria from the air plume downwind of a swine confined or concentrated animal feeding operation. *Environmental Health Perspectives*, 114(7), 1032-1037.]. This type of exposure can also make us sick. Recall that certain animal flu viruses may swap genetic material and produce new variants capable of infecting humans. As it turns out, bacteria have been doing something similar since the beginning of time. Many exchange pieces of DNA with largely unrelated bacterial species through the shedding and uptake of DNA fragments called plasmids. These small loops of DNA may include the key to antibiotic resistance and be shed from a relatively benign swine bacterium, incapable of infecting a human. But the plasmids may be taken up by lethal human-infecting bacteria, thereby bestowing antibiotic resistance to the human pathogen. Where once a shot of penicillin might have cured a person infected with such bacteria, now doctors must resort to ever more powerful and side effect–prone new antibiotics. And in some cases, no antibiotic, new or old, will work.

Overcrowding

Modern living also depresses immunity. For the first time in history, there are more people living in cities than anywhere else. Having higher numbers of people in concentrated areas leads to more pathogens and a greater strain on the immune system— not to mention a more dramatic and faster spread of communicable sickness [Sclar, E. D., Garau, P., & Carolini G. (2005). The 21st century health challenge of slums and cities. *Lancet*, 365(9462), 901-903.]. Adding to this immune burden is the fact that we are now a global planet; people travel faster than ever before, with air travel available to more people than ever before. With these travelers come germs. Illnesses that may have been found only in one place can now rapidly go global. The result is a much greater need to defend against diseases that were once distant and exotic.

Chronic Heightened Stress

Further, the day-to-day stresses that so many of us struggle with can also alter immunity and increase risk of illness. The fast pace of modern living mimics the flight or fight response, many times resulting in emotions like unfounded fear and a chronic anxious state. These result in the excessive release of cortisol and adrenocorticotropic hormone (ACTH), which lowers the immune response, reduces the amount of immune defender cells in tissues, and depresses the immune system's communication network [Martini, F. H. (2006). *Fundamentals of Anatomy and Physiology*. (7th Ed.). Toronto, Canada: Pearson Benjamin Cummings.].

5

OLIVE LEAF, ARABINOGALACTAN, AND ANDROGRAPHIS

YOUR IMMUNITY SOLUTION

Clearly, the immune system is vital to our very survival, and our modern world's immune-altering impact is a serious problem. Thankfully, research has uncovered a host of valuable nutrients, available in supplement form, that enhance and support immune function without side effects. While there are many natural supplements that help support healthy immune system performance, olive leaf, arabinogalactan, and andrographis are three of the best. Like a closely guarded secret, this trifecta of immune-supporting botanical nutrients is not as well-known as it should be. But it is quickly gaining ground. This book reveals what these supplements are, how they work, why they work, and how to take them.

Olive tree products, including olive leaf, have been a staple of Mediterranean medicine and cuisine for centuries. A powerful infection fighter, olive leaf extract has been shown to help eliminate bacteria, fungi, viruses (such as colds and flu), yeasts (like Candida), and parasites (such as the type that cause malaria). Olive leaf is used widely in Russia, Turkey, Greece, Italy, and throughout the Balkan countries. As you will see in the chapter devoted to olive leaf, studies have reported that olive leaf can positively affect cardiovascular health, high blood pressure, arthritis, cholesterol levels, and even cancer, in addition to its immune-supporting properties.

Arabinogalactan is a substance found in many plants, but especially in the Western larch tree (*Larix occidentalis*), which grows in British Columbia, Canada, and throughout the Pacific and Inland Northwest of the United States. In addition to the fact that it is a form of digestive-health–supporting fiber, arabinogalactan plays a role in supporting the immune system. Arabinogalactan increases the number of infection-fighting cells while, at the same time, supporting the good bacteria (or "friendly flora") found in the gut. Antibiotics destroy not only the bad bacteria, but also the friendly flora, leading to potential health complications such as yeast infections. When used as a preventive measure, arabinogalactan supplementation can bolster your immune defenses and strengthen the friendly flora in the GI tract. You could almost consider this immune maintenance for your body. If your immune system is able to fend off the common bugs during cold and flu season there is less need to enter into the excessive cycle of antibiotic use, which is all too common in our culture.

Andrographis paniculata is a plant with many names that has remained a vital part of health care and disease prevention throughout Asia for centuries. This plant contains active constituents, including andrographolides, that promote immune function, reduce fever, and combat many infectious diseases. It is widely used in Scandinavia to reduce the duration, symptoms, and severity of the cold and flu. It has been studied extensively and proven to be effective in reducing fever, decreasing inflammation, and boosting the immune system. This herb is one of the first things that I turn to at LaValle Metabolic Institute whenever someone has an upper respiratory infection or feels a cold coming on. Its results are always impressive.

Olive leaf extract, larch arabinogalactan, and *Andrographis paniculata* extract can be used to help your immune system achieve a heightened state of readiness, giving your immune system the upper hand the next time the cold, flu, or bacterial infections attempt an attack.

6

OLIVE LEAF
(*OLEA EUROPAEA*)

A CLOSER LOOK AT THE WORLD'S OLDEST AND MOST HONORED HERBAL MEDICINE

While most of us visualize the olive tree bearing its fruit—young green olives or ripe dark olives—the tree, which blooms with small white flowers, is prized for far more than its fruit.

BACKGROUND

Olive trees can easily reach 600 years of age—some existing olive trees are purported to be over 2000 years old—and still produce fruit. The trees grow in warmer climates, such as the Mediterranean, South Africa, Australia, California, New Zealand, Chile, Northwest Africa, and Israel. There are thousands of varieties of olive trees, all of which grow very slowly. The Mediterranean region is perhaps most strongly associated with the olive tree; its cultures have used the wood, leaves, and fruit of the olive tree for thousands of years, and notably have a lower incidence of heart disease and other chronic health conditions.

Mankind as a whole has an even longer history with the olive tree. Human consumption of olives began long ago. While people are believed to have consumed olives for tens of thousands of years, some archaeologists estimate that mankind has been actively cultivating olive trees for over 4000 years. Archaeological records also show that Egyptian olive trees were cultivated at least as far back as 500 BC and that northwestern Mediterranean trees had been cultivated during the early Bronze Age, and quite likely before that. Cultivation of the olive tree has led to over 900 different types of olives.

When it comes to the health-promoting properties of olive leaf, references extend back to early history. Ancient Egyptians were among the first to recognize the olive tree's potential medicinal applications. In fact, they regarded olive leaf with such reverence that they used its oil in the mummification of pharaohs and royalty.

The olive leaf's lofty reputation may extend to early Christianity as well. An intriguing Biblical passage quotes God describing a "tree of life" that could be a reference to the olive tree: "The fruit thereof shall be for meat, and the leaf thereof for medicine." In the book of Revelations, another "tree of life" reference reveals that "the leaves of the tree were for the healing of all nations." Given the many benefits of the olive leaf, this Biblical passage may very well be referring to the olive tree and its health-promoting leaves.

Ancient Greeks also held the olive tree in high esteem. The Goddess Athena was believed to have planted the very first olive tree, bestowing it with numerous mystical powers, including many related to health, such as curing sickness, healing wounds, and offering nourishing sustenance. Olive branches took on special significance in Greek culture. Woven into a wreath, the olive tree branches became *kotinos*—the crown awarded to Olympic champions. Olive oil was the original fuel for the Olympic torch.

HOW DOES IT WORK?

Though the true origins of its traditional healing properties are likely lost in the mist of history, olive leaf's emergence in modern medicine is dated around the mid-19th Century, when its anti-inflammatory capacity and ability to treat infections were both noticed.

By the early 20th Century, scientists had identified oleuropein, a bitter compound, as the "active ingredient" within olive leaf. Subsequent research of elenolic acid, a compound found within olive leaf's oleuropein, revealed findings that were nothing short of miraculous. Researchers' in vitro tests revealed that calcium elenolate, a derivative of elenolic acid, effectively wiped out a range of pathogens. Elenolate was found to be effective against a range of parasites and bacteria, including highly recognizable strains such as staph, salmonella,

E. coli, and malaria. Elenolate also appeared to fight off a number of health-threatening viruses, including those associated with influenza; parainfluenza; upper and lower respiratory tract infections; herpes; polio; and hand, foot, and mouth disease.

With effectiveness against such a broad range of insidious pathogens, olive leaf represented a remarkable health and immunity breakthrough. But how exactly does olive leaf do it? Researchers have suggested that the following mechanisms of the compounds found in olive leaf may account for its ability to promote peak immune system performance and support overall health: [Renis, HE. In vitro antiviral activity of calcium elenolate. *Antimicrobe Agents Chemother.*, 16-172 (1970).]

- Shuts down viruses, deprives them of "building blocks" for replication, and prevents them from spreading. Some of this anti-viral activity involves identifying sick cells and targeting viruses within them.

- Neutralizes free radical damage with powerful antioxidant activity. Antioxidants like those found in olive leaf have been shown to enhance many different immune system activities [Alvarado C, Alvarez P, Puerto M, Gausseres N, Jimenez L, De la Fuente M. Dietary supplementation with antioxidants improves functions and decreases oxidative stress of leukocytes from prematurely aging mice. *Nutrition*. 2006 Jul-Aug;22(7-8):767-77.].

- Promotes a healthy immune reaction by kick-starting *phagocytosis*, the process by which the immune system's defender cells engulf and destroy pathogens such as bacteria and parasites.

- Modulates the body's inflammatory response [Pieroni A, et al. In vitro anti-complementary activity of flavonoids from olive (*Olea europaea* L.) leaves. *Pharmazie*. Oct. 1996;51(10):765-8.]. Healthy inflammation is a marker of a well-tuned immune system.

With such extensive activity in the realm of immune system support, it's no surprise that olive leaf may offer numerous health benefits. By depriving bacteria and viruses of the building blocks they need to grow and replicate, olive leaf's oleuropein prevents infection from spreading enough to become noticeable. By triggering phagocytes into action, olive leaf increases the immune system's response to infection. Both of these steps are critical because illness manifests not when we absorb one virus, but when that virus succeeds in replicating and eliciting symptoms.

SCIENTIFIC EVIDENCE

Ongoing research has further reinforced olive leaf's ability to support the immune system and destroy harmful pathogens:

Olive Leaf as Antiviral

One study showed that olive leaf extract inhibited the infectivity of viral hemorrhagic septicemia virus (VHSV), a deadly fish virus that causes bleeding in muscles, internal organs, and other tissues. Researchers discovered that the oleuropein in olive leaf extract reduced the viral infectivity of VHSV by 30%—leading them to propose that olive leaf not only holds potential as a promising antiviral agent, but may be used as an example to design other antiviral agents [Micol V, Caturla N, Perez-Fons L, Mas V, Perez L, Estepa A. The olive leaf extract exhibits antiviral activity against viral haemorrhagic septicaemia rhabdovirus (VHSV) . Antiviral Res . 2005; 66:129-136.].

Olive Leaf as Antibacterial

Another study tested how secoridoides (oleuropein and derivatives) found in olives, olive leaf, and olive oil might fight pathogenic bacteria. The study examined five bacterial strains, including salmonella, along with 44 other isolates known to cause intestinal and respiratory tract infections. Both oleuropein and hydroxytyrosol, taken from olives, were found to exhibit significant antimicrobial activity—oleuropein was found to slow the growth of several bacteria strains, including the dreaded *E. coli* and *K. pneumoniae*. The researchers concluded that olive tree compounds might be considered a source of promising antimicrobial agents for treatment of intestinal or respiratory tract infections

[Bisignano, G, et al. On the in-vitro antimicrobial activity of oleuropein and hydroxytyrosol. *J Pharm Pharmacol* 1999 Aug; 51(8):971-4]. That study echoed the findings of an earlier study, which revealed that olive leaf extract is even effective against antibiotic-resistant and potentially life-threatening Staphylococcus aureus bacteria [Tranter HS, Tassou SC, Nychas GJ. (1993). The effect of the olive phenolic compound, oleuropein, on growth and enterotoxin B production by Staphylococcus aureus. *Applied Bacteriology*, 74, 253-259.].

Olive Leaf as Anti-HIV

Yet another impressive and significant testament to oleuropein's antiviral activity is its efficacy against HIV (human immunodeficiency virus). One study found that oleuropein blocked HIV transmission from cell to cell and also inhibited HIV replication [Lee-Huang S, Zhang L, Huang PL, Chang YT, Huang PL. Anti-HIV activity of olive leaf extract (OLE) and modulation of host cell gene expression by HIV-1 infection and OLE treatment. *Biochem Biophys Res Commun.* 2003; 307:1029-1037.].

Olive Leaf as Anti-Cancer

Olive leaf's oleuropein appears to reduce cancer cells' ability to reproduce, invade other cells, and travel to set up in other parts of the body. It may also inhibit cancerous tumors' ability to spread by blocking the formation of blood vessels to supply the tumor with nutrients, as well as preventing the cancerous cells from sticking to each other and anchoring themselves within the body. In this way, olive leaf extract may reduce the incidence and spread of cancers [Waterman, E., & Lockwood, B. Active components and clinical applications of olive oil. *Alternative Medicine Review*, 12(4), 331-342.].

A study performed in 1986 sparked much more investigation into olive leaf extract and specifically oleuropein. When researchers examined both the death rates and causes of death of Mediterranean people, who live with an abundance of olive trees nearby and consume olive tree products regularly, made an amazing discovery: these populations had a lower incidence of breast, skin, and colon cancer [Keys, A., Menotti, A., Karvonen, M. J, et al., (1986). The diet and 15 year death rate in the seven countries study. *American Journal of Epidemiology*, 124, 903-915.].

In 2005, a study was performed in which mice with cancerous tumors were given 1% oleuropein in their drinking water. The oleuropein not only stopped the cancer cells' ability to reproduce, travel, and invade other areas, but also shrank the tumor in 9-12 days [Hamdi K., Castellon R. Oleuropein, a non-toxic olive iridoid, is an anti-tumor agent and cytoskeleton disruptor. *Biochemical and Biophysical Research Communication*, 334(3), 769-778.].

A 2007 study reinforced the idea that oleuropein might slow cancer growth. In this study, breast cancer cells exposed to the various phyto-chemicals found in olive oil reproduced and spread less when oleuropein was administered than when any other component was used. [Menendez, J. et al., (2007). Olive oil's bitter principle reverses autoresistance to trastuzumab (Herceptin) in HER2-overexpressing breast cancer cells. *BMC Cancer,* 7(1), 80.].

Olive Leaf and Heart Health

A powerful antioxidant, olive leaf is believed to decrease oxidation of "bad" (LDL) cholesterol. When LDL cholesterol oxidizes, it can lead to dangerous artery damage, progression of plaque, and promotion of atherosclerosis, or narrowing of the arteries. Olive leaf is also believed to inhibit the platelet "clumping" that precedes blood clots that can cause stroke and heart attack. Researchers have hailed olive leaf as a natural botanical that lowers high blood pressure, lowers cholesterol levels, and helps to prevent heart disease [Waterman, E., & Lockwood, B. Active components and clinical applications of olive oil. *Alternative Medicine Review*, 12(4), 331-342.].

Olive Leaf and Rheumatoid Arthritis

Inflammation and immunity go hand in hand. Evidence suggests that olive leaf, by modulating inflammation and supporting healthy immune function, may hold benefits for those suffering from autoimmune disease and chronic inflammation.

Research indicates that oleuropein in particular possesses inflammation-modulating activity that may interfere with the chain of events that leads to chronic rheumatoid arthritis (RA). This effect could also be due to the fact that olive leaf has such strong antimicrobial action. Most people are unaware that many patients suffering from RA have excessive growth of harmful bacteria.

One study examining the benefits of fish oils for RA used olive oil as a placebo. Upon analyzing the results, researchers were surprised to find how much the group taking olive oil (which contains lesser amounts of oleuropein than the leaves) showed improvement [Kremer, J. M., Lawrence, D. A., Jubiz, W. et al., (1990). Dietary fish oil and olive oil supplementation in patients with rheumatoid arthritis. Clinical and immunologic effects. *Arthritis Rheumatoid*, 33, 810-820.]. Another scientific study showed that exposure of human blood cultures to oleuropein was associated with a staggering 80% decrease in inflammatory chemicals [Miles, E. A., Zoubouli, P., & Calder, P. C. (2005). Differential anti-inflammatory effects of phenolic compounds from extra virgin olive oil identified in human whole blood cultures. *Nutrition*, 21(3), 389-394], while a scientific literature review cited oleuropein as a natural anti-inflammatory agent capable of benefiting health [Patrick L., Uzick M. Cardiovascular Disease: C-Reactive Protein and the Inflammatory Disease Paradigm: HMG-CoA

Reductase Inhibitors, alpha-Tocopherol, Red Yeast Rice, and Olive Oil Polyphenols. A Review of the Literature. *Alternative Medicine Review*, June, 2001.]. Considering the extensive negative health complications associated with chronic inflammation, olive leaf's inflammation-modulating activity may help to support immune function and overall well-being in more ways than we can imagine.

What does olive leaf's multifaceted impact on human health all add up to? Olive leaf proponent Dr. Morton Walker may have said it best when he proclaimed olive leaf to be "the one true, natural, and non-toxic way to eliminate illnesses arising from viruses, bacteria, fungi, yeasts, protozoa, worms, flukes, and other parasites. Ingredients in olive leaves work against those specific microbes causing herpes infections, skin diseases, candidiasis, malaria, arthritis, heart trouble, flu and even the common cold." [Walker, M. (1999). Olive leaf extract. *Better Nutrition*, 61(4), 38.]. Walker also reported that olive leaf lessens the symptoms of fibromyalgia, chronic fatigue, Lyme disease, yeast infections, athlete's foot and jock itch. With this diverse mixed-bag of health benefits, olive leaf appears a truly amazing health tonic supplied by nature.

HOW IS IT TAKEN?

For general purpose immune support, I recommend a good quality supplement providing

250 mg olive leaf, standardized to 6% oleuropein, per day.

However, oftentimes people need a little more than this basic, general support regimen (for example, to rid yourself of the tail end of annoying cold symptoms, or to take along on a ski trip, knowing that your system will be stressed by the elements). In such cases, I recommend something a bit stronger, such as 500 mg of olive leaf extract standardized to 6% oleuropein, or, for a little stronger response, 250 mg standardized to 20% oleuropein per day.

In cases where I am combating a common cold that's running through a family or an office environment, I sometimes recommend an even stronger level, such as 250 mg standardized 20%, twice daily.

The good thing about standardized olive leaf supplements is that they come in many different dosage levels and delivery forms, such as capsules, tablets and extended release (or extended delivery) tablets. This provides great flexibility for adapting dosages to an individual's particular needs.

Standardization—as measured by testing—assures that batches of the supplement maintain a consistent amount of an ingredient, which assures potency from batch to batch. The Considerations section describes the importance of standardization in greater detail.

I have given you the information you need to take olive leaf by itself. But before you run out to buy a bottle of olive leaf extract, be sure to read the Considerations section, which addresses taking olive leaf in combination with arabinogalactans and andrographis, for even better results.

7

LARCH ARABINOGALACTAN (*LARIX OCCIDENTALIS*) (ARA-LARIX)

THE WORLD'S MOST EFFECTIVE IMMUNE-BOOSTING FIBER

Arabinogalactan is a phytochemical, or natural chemical component, of many plants. Arabinogalactan exists as a polysaccharide (a string of simple sugars) in such plants as carrots, pears, tomatoes, and radishes.

BACKGROUND

The greatest concentration of arabinogalactan is found in the wood of the Western larch (*Larix occidentalis*) tree; in fact, the powder extracted from the larch tree contains approximately 98% arabinogalactan. In this book we'll refer to arabinogalactan as ARA-Larix, since Western larch arabinogalactan is the source most found in dietary supplements.

ARA-Larix is a powerful agent for the elimination and prevention of bacterial and viral infections, working on two fronts:

1. ARA-Larix promotes healthy elimination and a healthy gastrointestinal function.

ARA-Larix is recognized as a good source of dietary fiber, so its most obvious role (from a biochemical point of view) would be to support the health of the gastrointestinal tract. And, like most forms of dietary fiber, ARA-Larix supports cardiovascular health by inhibiting low-density lipid absorption. Yet, unlike most forms of dietary fiber, the activity of ARA-Larix is not limited to either of these activities.

2. ARA-Larix places the immune system in a continual state of peak performance to identify and eliminate invading organisms.

The primary reason for taking ARA-Larix is for its powerful immune-boosting capacity. ARA-Larix has been shown to be more a potent enhancer of the immune response than even the benchmark botanical, echinacea. Yet, you can take ARA-Larix as a long-term agent to keep the immune system at peak performance. You can take ARA-Larix daily for months, without the fear that the body will build up a tolerance and thereby diminish its effectiveness. And, since ARA-Larix is a completely different form of phytonutrient from olive leaf, echinacea, goldenseal, astragalus, and others, ARA-Larix and extracts of these immune-supportive herbs can be taken together for a compounded effect.

This minimizes the chance of overloading any single aspect of immune response because it promotes multiple and separate immune pathways.

HOW DOES IT WORK?

ARA-Larix was approved by the U.S. Food and Drug Administration as a good way to increase dietary fiber to support digestive health, but it has since exhibited additional health-promoting properties—most notably, it stimulates the immune system.

One theory on just how ARA-Larix works comes from clues obtained through investigations into bacteria and fungi. These and other forms of infectious microbial invaders create a coating around themselves; this coating actually contains arabinogalactan-like molecules and other closely related compounds. It is believed that the human immune system may be evolutionarily tuned to keep an eye out for the presence of such substances, as they indicate the threat of a microbial infection. Once detected, the immune system responds to arabinogalactan with extra production of antibodies and other defensive elements because it believes it is sensing the production of arabinogalactan in the cell walls of bacteria and fungi.

The accompanying graph displays the results of a study comparing the ability of ARA-Larix to enhance macrophage proliferation versus that of echinacea. The differences between these two botanical extracts are plainly visible. Echinacea's effects appear to increase as the dose of echinacea extract becomes stronger. But it appears to peak at a specific level (100 mcg/ml in the blood), after which the concentration of defensive macrophages drops back down to its originally low levels.

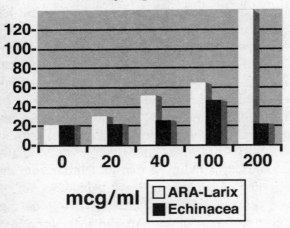

These results indicate that the maximum output of protective macrophages one can attain through echinacea supplementation occurs at a specific level. More echinacea becomes less effective. ARA-Larix supplementation, on the other hand, exhibits no such peak followed by ineffective levels. As the chart indicates, supplementation with ARA-Larix enhances macrophage proliferation nearly twice as effectively as echinacea supplementation does.

Research suggests that ARA-Larix is involved in many different facets of immune function, as listed below [Kelly, GS. Larch Arabinogalactan: Clinical relevance of a novel immune-enhancing polysaccharide. *Alternative Medicine Review*. 1999; Vol. 4, No. 2, pp 96-103.]:

1. **Activates phagocytosis**. Phagocytosis is the process by which the immune system's cells engulf and dispose of harmful pathogens.

2. **Boosts the immune system's natural killer cell production.** This occurs as a result of increased secretion of chemicals (interleukin 2 and gamma interferon) which increase natural killer cell activity [Bouic, P. J. D. (2007). Plant sterols/sterolins for optimum immunity. *Positive Health*. 133, 32-35.]. Natural killer cells find and destroy abnormal tissue cells, and are especially important in the prevention of cancer. Different types of cancers can decrease natural killer cell activity; therefore, some experts believe ARA-Larix may hold potential to help suppress and interfere with the progression of certain cancers. [Hagmar B, et al. Arabinogalactan Blockade of Experimental Metastases to Liver by Murine Hepatoma. *Invasion Metastasis*. 1991;11:348-355.].

3. **Potentiates the activity of the reticuloendothelial system (RES).** Part of the immune system, the RES refers to phagocytic cells including macrophages and monocytes. These

cells are a class of those amoeba-like white blood cells I described in Chapter 2, produced in bone marrow.

4. **Promotes growth of friendly intestinal flora such as bifidobacteria and lactobacillus.** Recent supermarket trends reflect the importance of probiotics, or friendly flora; many food items boast that they contain "active cultures" of friendly flora. As described at the end of Chapter 2, these bacteria are needed for optimal immune system function and help to regulate immune performance. They also help the body to absorb vital nutrients, cleanse and detoxify the body, defend against and help to ward off inflammatory bowel disorders. These organisms ferment the ARA-Larix and use it as food; therefore, ARA-Larix may be considered a pre-biotic [Robinson, R. R., Feirtag, J., & Slavin, J. L. (2001). Effects of dietary arabinogalactan on gastrointestinal and blood parameters in healthy human subjects. *Journal of the American College of Nutrition*, 20(4), 279-285.].

5. **Neutralizes bacteria.** Once ingested, ARA-Larix polysaccharides prevent harmful microorganisms from replicating.

6. **Increases production of short-chain fatty acids.** One of these short-chain fatty acids, butyrate, has been shown to interfere with colon cancer cell growth [Augeron, C. & Laboisse, C. L. (1984) Emergence of permanently differentiated

cell clones in a human colonic cancer cell line after treatment with sodium butyrate. *Cancer Res.* 44: 3961–3969.] and is associated with a decreased incidence of colon cancer [Okata, M., Singhal, A. & Hakomori, S. (1989) Antibody-mediated targeting of differentiation inducers to tumor cells: inhibition of colonic cancer cell growth in vivo and in vitro. *Biochem. Biophys. Res. Commun.* 158: 202–208.]. Additionally, short-chain fatty acids are an important energy source, and enable the body to better absorb important minerals including calcium, magnesium, and iron [Hara Hiroshi, Physiological effects of short-chain fatty acid produced from prebiotics in the colon. *Bioscience and microflora.* 2002, vol. 21.].

7. **Decreases ammonia production.** Ammonia is toxic to the body and can have negative health consequences; excessive ammonia in the body is associated with serious illnesses such as Reye's Syndrome. Those with poor-functioning or damaged kidneys and liver—organs that filter ammonia and remove it—are especially at risk for ammonia toxicity.

SCIENTIFIC EVIDENCE

Scores of studies have given larch arabinogalactan a sort of cult following among researchers and natural healthcare practitioners. Gregory S. Kelly, respected Doctor of Naturopathy and noted nutritional researcher, stated in a published review of larch arabinogalactan, "Experimental studies have indicated larch arabinogalactan can stimulate natural killer (NK) cell [a form of white blood cell] cytotoxicity [ability to kill invading pathogens], enhance other functional aspects of the immune system, and inhibit the metastasis of tumor cells to the liver." [Kelly GS, Larch arabinogalactan: clinical relevance of a novel immune-enhancing polysaccharide. *Altern Med Rev.* 1999 Apr;4(2):96-103.] And numerous other researchers have described additional benefits. Here, you will see what the research studies say about the health-boosting effects of ARA-Larix.

More Friendly Bacteria

In a 2001 randomized, placebo-controlled, double-blind study, adult participants were given 15g or 30g of ARA-Larix for three weeks, and then crossed over to the other dose for an additional three weeks. At the end of the study, researchers found that taking ARA-Larix orally resulted in increased numbers of friendly flora, specifically Lactobacillus. Researchers found this outcome to be significant because Lactobacilli destroy toxins, produce antimicrobial compounds, and maintain and restore intestinal balance [Pfeifer A, Rosat JP: Probiotics in alimentation; clinical evidence for their enhancement of the natural immunity of the gut. In Hanson, Yolken (eds): "Probiotics, Other Nutritional Factors, and Intestinal

Microflora." Philadelphia: Lippencott-Raven, 1999.].
Some species of Lactobacilli may also possess
immune-regulating activity, including boosting phagocytosis in the blood. In addition to bolstering friendly
flora, the study found that ARA-Larix decreased participants' ammonia levels. Notably, ARA-Larix's beneficial effects in this study were present in both the
15g group and the 30g group [Robinson, R. R.,
Feirtag, J., & Slavin, J. L. (2001). Effects of dietary
arabinogalactan on gastrointestinal and blood parameters in healthy human subjects. *Journal of the
American College of Nutrition*, 20(4), 279-285).].

Fewer Ear Infections in Children

Clinical evidence published in 1996 showed that
healthy children who were given ARA-Larix on a
regular basis had far fewer ear infections than a
group of children who did not take ARA-Larix
[D'Adamo, P. (1996). Larch arabinogalactan.
Journal of Naturopathic Medicine, 6, 33-37.].

Enhanced Natural Defenses Against Chronic Conditions

Many diseases are characterized by lowered
amounts of natural killer cells, including chronic
fatigue syndrome, HIV, multiple sclerosis, and
hepatitis (both B and C). ARA-Larix's ability to
increase the number and activity of natural killer
cells, as well as other white blood cells involved in
immunity, suggests that it may hold promise as an
adjunctive therapeutic agent to be used alongside

treatment for conditions marked by diminished natural killer cell counts [D'Adamo, P. (1996). Larch arabinogalactan. *Journal of Naturopathic Medicine*, 6, 33-37.].

Protection from Cancer

ARA-Larix's promising potential as a cancer therapy is garnering a buzz in the natural health arena. In one especially exciting animal study, ARA-Larix appeared to slow the progression of cancer. In the study, administering ARA-Larix significantly reduced the number of liver metastases, while simultaneously prolonging survival [Hagmar B, Ryd W, Skomedal H. Arabinogalactan blockade of experimental metastases to liver by murine hepatoma. *Invasion Metastasis* 1991;11:348-355.]. Metastases are instances in which cancer cells have broken free of the confines of the tissue from which they originated, more simply known as the devastating "spread" of cancer.

These findings were especially relevant because metastatic cancerous cells typically spread to the liver first. When considered alongside other reports that suggest ARA-Larix may stimulate natural killer cells and inhibit cancer cells from reproducing and spreading, these results offer a glimmer of hope that natural botanicals like ARA-Larix may someday help to conquer cancer [Kelly GS. Larch arabinogalactan: clinical relevance of a novel immune-enhancing polysaccharide. *Altern Med Rev.* 4, 2:96-103, 1999.].

HOW IS IT TAKEN?

ARA-Larix is generally taken orally as a supplement, usually made from powdered soluble and odorless fiber of the larch tree. Typically, 1000-3000 mg of ARA-Larix is taken for immune enhancement, specifically targeted against a particular condition. For example, when a cold or flu virus is spreading throughout the office (targeted prevention). As I discussed in the chapter on olive leaf, standardization affects the amount of active ingredients. Current literature indicates that supplements should be 98% arabinogalactan. The dosage suggested for an acute condition is 500 mg, two to four times a day for 7–10 days. For chronic illness, targeted prevention, and immune support, consider using it three weeks on, one week off. When in doubt, read the labels carefully and talk to a nutritionist or naturopathic doctor for the best advice.

8

ANDROGRAPHIS PANICULATA

THE WORLD'S MOST EFFECTIVE ANTI-FLU IMMUNE BOOSTER

Andrographis paniculata, known as Maha-tita', or "king of bitters," has been a key component in Ayurveda, the ancient Indian healing science, for thousands of years. Recently, modern researchers have validated many Ayurvedic practices, including the use of andrographis.

BACKGROUND

A rediscovery of such ancient uses, as well as modern scientific substantiation, have propelled andrographis to the top of the therapeutic supplements market. From relative obscurity just a few short years ago, *Andrographis paniculata* has become one of the fastest growing herbal immune-supporting supplements. The entire plant is believed to have healing qualities; even its roots are valued for their medicinal properties. Typically though, it is the leaves and stems (aerial parts) that are harvested at the end of summer for their immune system boosting properties.

A foundation herb of Traditional Chinese Medicine, andrographis is known as Chuan Xin Lian, a "cold" herb that helps the body detoxify and disperse excessive heat. In Traditional Chinese and Indian Ayurvedic medical practices, andrographis is highly regarded for its ability to ease pain, as well as for its positive impact on liver and digestive health. Ayurvedic traditions and modern medicine agree that when digestion is healthy, the immune system's response will be more robust— good digestive health is often an indicator of andrographis' (or any medicinal herb's) immune-strengthening properties.

Andrographis has been used for hundreds of years against malaria, diarrhea, herpes, bronchitis, cholera, parasites, gonorrhea, upper respiratory infections, sore throat, and numerous other health problems. Andrographis is also used in Scandinavian countries, where it enjoys tremendous popularity as a remedy for the common cold. Though historically andrographis has been most recognized for its support of digestive health and positive influence on liver activity and detoxification, its ability to modulate inflammation and boost the immune system is largely responsible for its current popularity.

Though it may seem like a new herb to our Western culture, andrographis has an impressive history of immune support. In fact, medicinal use of andrographis is credited with halting the progression of the 1919 flu epidemic in India.

HOW DOES IT WORK?

Though andrographis is rich in many different inflammation-modulating flavonoids, modern science has identified andrographolides as the herb's most active ingredients. These phytochemicals, which are most concentrated in the leaves, are extremely bitter; in fact, some traditions judge the plant's medicinal efficacy by how bitter it tastes.

Andrographis is rapidly absorbed by the body and incorporated into the bloodstream shortly after it is taken. Then, andrographolides tend to migrate to the spleen, among other organs. One of the primary roles of the spleen is to house lymphocytes, which are a kind of white blood cell that help the body fight off infection. In fact, people who have had their spleens removed are generally at greater risk for infections. The presence of andrographolides in the spleen may help explain part of its role in supporting immunity.

Andrographis is believed to stimulate both nonspecific immune responses and antigen-specific immune responses. The nonspecific immune response is our first line of defense that rallies to protect the body when it is invaded by a new pathogen for the first time. Antigen-specific immune response is our second line of defense, which takes action when nonspecific immune responses fail. Additionally, antigen-specific immunity is the part that "remembers" past encounters with pathogens. Andrographis also appears to support immunity in the following ways [Barilla, J. (1999). *Andrographis paniculata*. Better Nutrition, 61(6), 26.]:

- Boosts production of white blood cells, which go on to devour pathogens.
- Enables release of interferon, a powerful hormone-like signaling protein that helps destroy viruses and prevent them from replicating.
- Enhances performance of white blood cells, improving their ability to recognize and eliminate pathogens [Ji LL, et al. Andrograpanin, a compound isolated from anti-inflammatory traditional Chinese medicine, *Andrographis paniculata*, enhances chemokine SDF-1 alpha induced leukocytes chemotaxis. *J Cell Biogem*, 2005 Aug 1; 95(5) 970-8.].
- Supports activity of the entire lymph system.
- Triggers the body's natural production of antibodies and macrophages—helping to bolster the body's defenses against a wide range of pathogens, bacteria, microbes, and cancer-causing agents [Puri, A., R. Saxena, R.P. Saxena, and K.C. Saxena. 1993. Immunostimulant agents from *Andrographis paniculata*. *J. Natural Products* 56(7):995-99.].

The significance of andrographis' legendary ability to reduce fevers and inflammation cannot be overstated. The immune system's macrophages, as mentioned earlier, act as a surveillance and security system, finding and removing threats like viruses. Macrophages also play a role in inflammation. For example, if we stub our toe, chemicals are released that start the process of inflammation. Macrophages are called to rush into the area through chemical signals to remove broken cells and other debris. Although our body has an amazing way of fixing damage, sometimes it overreacts, causing the immune response to generate excessive inflammation that over time can become very dangerous. Andrographis helps slow down the inflammatory macrophages, decreasing inflammation. In fact, one 2007 study reported that andrographis was such an effective anti-inflammatory that researchers concluded that it should be developed into a commercial anti-inflammatory preparation [Liu, J., Wang, Z., & Ji, L. (2007). In vivo and in vitro anti-inflammatory activities of neoandrographolide. *American Journal of Chinese Medicine, 35*(2), 317-328.].

What do these mechanisms all add up to? Modern science is revealing that andrographis possesses a miraculous ability to harmonize with our internal defenses, providing remarkably complex, multifaceted support for peak immune system performance. Andrographis appears to "tune" the immune system so that it reacts appropriately; boosting it when needed, but also ensuring that inflammation does not run rampant and damage the body. The ultimate result of this fine-tuning can be seen in the well-designed clinical trials and analyses that validate andrographis' role as one of the most important immune-supporting botanicals ever discovered.

SCIENTIFIC EVIDENCE

Colds, sore throats, sniffles, and influenza—what if there were a substance that could not only ease upper respiratory infections' symptoms and hasten recovery, but also prevent such infections from occurring altogether? An ever-growing body of scientific evidence suggests that andrographis might do just that.

First, consider the big picture: meta-analyses. While meta-analyses have their shortcomings, when conducted properly, this type of investigation can have value. They choose the best-designed studies, gather them together, and then draw conclusions based upon a large pool of data. One such meta-analysis combined seven double blind controlled trials (very rigorous), totaling 896 subjects, that investigated andrographis' medicinal efficacy in the treatment of upper respiratory infections. The collected data found that andrographis is superior to placebo in reducing upper respiratory tract infection symptoms, and may even have a preventive effect [Coon JT, Ernst E. *Andrographis paniculata* in the treatment of upper respiratory tract infections: a systematic review of safety and efficacy. *Planta Med* 2004;70:293-8.].

A systematic review of three randomized, controlled trials analyzed andrographis' impact on 433 total patients. The researchers concluded that andrographis appears to be an appropriate alternative treatment of upper respiratory tract infection, whether it is used alone or in conjunction with Siberian Ginseng (eleuthero) [Poolsup N, Suthisisang C, Prathanturarug S, et al. *Andrographis paniculata* in the symptomatic treatment of uncomplicated upper respiratory tract infection: systematic review of randomized controlled trials. *J Clin Pharm Ther* 2004;29:37-45.].

Additional stand-alone studies suggest that andrographis may ward off the common cold, hasten recovery from the cold, ease inflammation, and help alleviate symptoms like fever and sore throat:

- One randomized, placebo-controlled, double blind study examined men and women between 25 and 50 years of age suffering from a common cold. Half the patients received placebo; the other half received 1200 mg each day of an andrographis dried extract standardized to 5 mg of total andrographolide and deoxyandrographolide, the active ingredients of the herb. Patients were then tested at intervals for the impact andrographis had on symptoms. By the second day of the treatment, patients receiving andrographis exhibited significant reduction in the intensity of symptoms like runny nose, fatigue, and sore throat. By day 4, the intensity of all symptoms evaluated in the study, including sleeplessness and earache, had also significantly decreased. Researchers concluded that andrographis was highly effective in alleviating the symptoms of the common cold; a result attributed to the herb's potential as an immune-stimulating tonic [Caceres DD, et al. Use of visual analogue scale measurements to assess the effectiveness of standardized *Andrographis paniculata* extract SHA-10 in reducing the symptoms of the common cold. A randomized double blind placebo study. *Phytomedicine*, Vol 6, 1999, pp 217-223.].

- A randomized, double blind study also found that andrographis might help people avoid catching colds altogether. In the study, 107 volunteers, all around age 18, were split into two groups that received either placebo or a Scandinavian product that features standardized extract of *Andrographis paniculata*. Participants took their tablets for five days a week over the course of three winter months, and were evaluated weekly by a clinician for any signs of the common cold. By month three the andrographis group exhibited a significant decrease in common cold incidence. Overall, at study's end, the andrographis group was found to have experienced a 50% reduction in risk for catching cold [Caceres, DD, et al. Prevention of common colds with *Andrographis paniculata* dried extract. A pilot double blind trial. *Phytomedicine*, 1997 Vol 4 (2), pp. 101-104.].

- A 1999 pilot study measured the effectiveness of an andrographis extract versus conventional treatment for influenza in 540 patients aged 19-63. The herbal nutrition group took a standardized extract of andrographis (88.8 mg) and eleuthero (10.0 mg) for 3–5 days. During physician visits, patients' symptoms—fever, cough, headaches, body aches, and other usual suspects—were recorded. After the study analysis ended, researchers concluded that the group that took andrographis extract recovered faster and were less likely to suffer from post-influenza complications [Kulichenko LL, Kireyeva LC, Malayshkina EN, Wikman G. A randomized controlled study of Kan Jang versus Amantadine in the treatment of influenza in Volgograd. *J Herbal Pharmacother*. 2003;3(1): 77-93.].

- A double blind study of 152 participants with fever and sore throats again revealed andrographis' alleviating effect on cold symptoms. Participants taking 6g of andrographis per day over a course of seven days were found to have enjoyed a reduction in sore throat and fever symptoms—the extent of which was found to be similar to that of taking acetaminophen [Thamlikitkul V, Dechatiwongse T, Theerapong S, et al. Efficacy of *Andrographis paniculata*

(Nees) for pharyngotonsillitis in adults. *J Med Assoc Thai*.1991;74:437-442.].

Andrographis presents a fascinating revelation: while drug companies have labored for decades to create an effective synthetic cold remedy, one of nature's brilliant creations—long-used in traditional and folk medicine—has been here to help us with colds and flu all along. With such solid scientific evidence backing its efficacy, we can see the end results of andrographis' ability to fine-tune the immune system and modulate the inflammatory response. This is no small achievement, since flu is one of the leading causes of death in the elderly and it is a significant reason for lost time at work in the United States. While these remarkable herbal properties are clearly effective against mild and moderate conditions in the cold and flu family, they may also help support the body's defense against far more serious conditions.

Andrographis and Cancer

Cancer can be defined as an out-of-control growth of cells that fail to mature properly. This is known as an undifferentiated cell. If a cancer cell can be signaled to mature properly—also known as "differentiation"—it can be reprogrammed to remember its function and characteristics. Once the reprogramming occurs, it triggers the process of apoptosis, otherwise known as programmed cell death. Compounds called terpenes found in andrographis have been found to be remarkably effective in stimulating differentiation in cancer cells, suggesting potential anti-cancer activity. Additionally, andrographolides—the "active ingredients" of the andrographis herb—possess cytotoxic properties: they kill cancer cells [Talukdar, P.B., and S. Banerjee. 1968. Studies on the stability of andrographolide. *Indian J. Chem.* 6:252-54.].

- One study isolated andrographolide and found that it inhibited the proliferation of different tumor cell lines, suggesting its efficacy in fighting a range of different cancer types. The researchers concluded that andrographolide exerts direct anticancer activity, possesses immune-modulating properties, and may have the potential to be developed into a cancer therapeutic agent. [Rajagopal, S., et al. Andrographolide, a potential cancer therapeutic agent isolated from *Andrographis paniculata*. *Journal of Experimental Therapeutics and Oncology* 3 (3), 147-158.].

- Yet another study found that andrographis appeared to interfere with tumor formation. This 2007 study gave mice that had cancerous tumors andrographis and isolated andrographolides. The result was startling: Administration of andrographis and andrographolides appeared to kick-start the immune system, increasing production of natural killer cells which then attacked the tumor cells. The researchers concluded that—in both healthy and tumor-bearing mice—andrographis and andrographolide administration could significantly enhance the production of bone marrow cells (including white blood cells used by the immune system), interleukin-2 (the immune system's signaling molecule), and interferon-{gamma} (a signaling molecule that tells macrophages to attack tumors) [Sheeja, K, et al. Modulation of natural killer cell activity, antibody-dependent cellular cytotoxicity, and antibody-dependent complement-mediated cytotoxicity by andrographolide in normal and Erlich ascites carcinoma-bearing mice. *Integrative Cancer Therapies*, 6(1), 66-73).].

If andrographis can help with a simple common cold and the complex devastation of cancer, imagine what it can do for everything in between. Andrographis clearly has an amazing history of multifaceted support for human health through support of the immune system and more. Modern science is now confirming many folk medicine andrographis applications, yielding surprising benefits. Published reports suggest that andrographis also may offer the following benefits:

• Destroys the herpes virus without harming normal cells [Wiart et al. (2005). Antiviral properties of ent-labdene diterpenes of *Andrographis paniculata* nees, inhibitors of herpes simplex virus type 1. *Phytotherapy Research*, 19(12), 1069-1070.].

- Possesses antiseptic properties [Grossberg, G. T., & Fox, B. (2007). *The Essential Herb-Drug-Vitamin Interaction Guide: The Safe Way to use Medications and Supplements Together.* New York: Broadway Books.].
- Serves as an anti-venom for snake bites [Samy, R.P., Thwin, M.M., Gopalakrishnakone, P., & Ignacimuthu, S. (2008). Ethnobotanical survey of folk plants for the treatment of snakebites in Southern part of Tamilnadu, India. *Journal of Ethnopharmacology,* 115(2), 302-312.] and scorpion stings [Uawonggul, N., Chaveerach, A., Thammasirirak, S., Arkaravichien, T., Chuachan, C., & Daduang, S. (2006). Screening of plants acting against Heterometrus loaticus scorpion venom activity on fibroblast cell lysis. *Journal of Ethnopharmacology,* 103(2), 201-207.].
- Stops diarrhea, lowers blood pressure, lowers blood sugar, reduces the risk of developing ulcers, protects the liver from toxins [Barilla, J. (1999). *Andrographis paniculata. Better Nutrition,* 61(6), 26.].

All these discoveries, as impressive as they are, may be simply opening the door a crack to more far-reaching herbal medicine applications for andrographis: It has also been found in in-vitro studies to interfere with the platelet clumping that precedes heart attacks and strokes, and has also been suggested to possess anti-HIV properties.

HOW IS IT TAKEN?

I often recommend andrographis supplements at 150 mg, standardized to 50% andrographolides for targeted prevention. As I've described in previous chapters, I use the term "targeted prevention" to refer to situations where one is attempting to target preventive measures against a bug that's going around; for example when a cold or flu virus is spreading throughout your office, and you don't want to be the next victim.

For acute situations, such as when you know you're coming down with something, I recommend 300 mg to 600 mg per day of andrographis, standardized to 50% andrographolides.

9

CONSIDERATIONS

The preceding chapters have given you a good roadmap to the use of olive leaf extract, larch arabinogalactan, and *Andrographis paniculata* extract. But there is much more to botanical immune-boosting therapy than simply knowing the plant, its active constituents, and a daily milligram quantity to take. For optimal results, it is best to not only use quality extractions of researched herbal supplements, but also to follow through consistently with changes in diet as well as lifestyle.

This chapter will offer useful, excellent advice for accomplishing both. Today, more than ever, many people are looking for ways to improve their health through changing the way they eat as well as the way they live. Others may realize that their schedules allow them to adopt only some of the optimizing strategies presented here. If you cannot adopt a healthier lifestyle, but still wish to achieve superior immune-boosting results, there are many parts of this chapter that will help you get the most out of the herbal supplements you use.

In addition to immune-enhancing lifestyle techniques, this chapter will provide information to help you choose the very best herbal supplements on the market. It will show you that all supplements are not created equal. With a basic understanding of a few hallmarks of supplement quality, you will discover that the best, most active botanical supplements are actually quite easy to find.

IMMUNE-ENHANCING LIFESTYLE TECHNIQUES

Proper nutrition may be the single most important factor when it comes to peak immune function. Unfortunately, few of us are getting the nutrition we need for overall health and well-being, let alone immune performance.

Nutrition

In this section I address:

- Olive leaf, arabinogalactan (ARA-Larix), and andrographis in combination.
- Vitamins and minerals important to immune function.
- Other healthful botanicals.

Olive Leaf, Arabinogalactan (ARA-Larix), and Andrographis In Combination

In each of the individual chapters covering olive leaf, arabinogalactan (ARA-Larix), and andrographis, I describe my recommendation for taking any of them individually. But the real power of these immune system-enhancers comes from combining the three of them. With each of them addressing a different area of your immune defenses, the effects are not only additive, but synergistic. Synergy means that you get a greater effect than you would expect from the sum of the parts. I recommend the following combination for its potency and versatility:

- Olive leaf extract at 250 mg standardized to 20%–25% oleuropein, and additionally standardized to 10 other olive leaf constituents;
- Western larch ARA-Larix 500 mg of arabinogalactan; and
- *Andrographis paniculata* extract at 150 mg, standardized to 75 mg andrographolides.

At these levels, such a combination botanical supplement can be taken at a single dose per day to boost general immune defenses and for targeted prevention. Individuals may wish to achieve such a robust immune boost when the threat of falling ill is greater. For example, when you expect to be in crowded or confined places (such as airplanes, buses, transportation terminals, etc.) or when you plan on attending a school play during cold and flu season, it is a good idea to preemptively fortify your immune defenses.

At twice the single-dose concentration per day, this level yields an even more powerful immune boost. And this is to be expected because it provides the active constituents of each of the three herbs at levels that are documented in a number of research studies. These levels are best for situations where you know that coming down with the cold, flu, sore throat, or other bug is imminent or has already started. These levels can make the difference between a seven-day bout with the cold and two or three days of sniffles.

Vitamins and Minerals

Boosting intake of the right vitamins and minerals is a critically important first step when it comes to achieving peak immune system performance:

- **B Vitamins:** Chronic stress depletes the body's B vitamin resources; deficiencies of B vitamins have been linked with fewer of the immune system's lymphocytes and T-cells (types of white blood cells).

- **Selenium:** This antioxidant is believed to enhance the activation, proliferation, and function of the immune system's lymphocytes and T-cells. Some evidence suggests that when the body is deficient in selenium, viruses mutate more easily, leading to illness that stick around longer and cause more damage.

- **Vitamin A:** Another key immune-supporting nutrient, vitamin A is necessary for the development of immune cells and is essential for adaptive immune reactions. When the body doesn't get enough vitamin A, white blood cells do not function as well, and are less empowered to defend against pathogens.

- **Vitamin C:** The most famous of the immune-supporting nutrients, vitamin C is a powerful antioxidant that neutralizes free radicals, increases white blood cell counts, boosts interferon, and elevates antibodies. Also recharges Vitamin E.

- **Zinc:** This mineral performs a diverse array of functions within the immune system; even a mild zinc deficiency has been linked to reduced production of lymphocytes.

Other Botanical Immune Boosters

In addition to vitamins and minerals, herbal and probiotic supplements can provide significant immune system support. Olive leaf, ARA-Larix, and andrographis are just the beginning—there are a whole host of additional botanicals with an impressive history of enhancing immune performance:

- **Astragalus:** This tonic herb, used in traditional Chinese Medicine, enhances immune function in a number of different ways. It is believed to help activate immune response, stimulate microphages, T-cells, and natural killer cells, and generally nudges stem cells (in bone marrow) to develop into specific types of immune defender cells.

- **Beta-Glucans:** Found in medicinal mushrooms, grains (including barley and oats), and some yeasts, these polysaccharides help launch defenses by activating macrophages, but also limit immune response by ensuring the system does not overreact to pathogen invaders. Beta-glucans may be the active ingredients behind traditional Chinese Medicine's long history of using medicinal mushrooms such as Maitake and Reishi for immune-related health problems.

- **Echinacea:** Like the Western larch, echinacea also contains arabinogalactan, although in much smaller concentration. Also known as the purple coneflower, echinacea is believed to stimulate phagocytosis, possess antibacterial properties, and generally enhance the immune system's performance. Echinacea's efficacy is supported by its large, loyal following of users, making it one of the best-selling herbal supplements for immune support.

- **Elderberry:** Known for its soothing effect on cold and flu sufferers, the elderberry is rich in antioxidants and is believed to boost immune function by elevating production of cellular communication molecules and regulating the immune response.

- **Probiotics:** These friendly bacteria, available in supplement form, are useful for inhibiting the growth of "bad" bacteria, restoring the internal balance of intestinal microflora, promoting healthy digestion, and supporting peak immune system function. It is particularly important to consume probiotics after finishing a round of antibiotics. That's because antibiotics do not discriminate; they destroy the good bacteria along with the bad. A big challenge in purchasing probiotics is finding one that retains good viability at the shelf. Probiotics must be alive in order to be useful. Unfortunately, probiotic microorganisms do not survive all environments and potential temperature variations. Poor temperature and humidity control during the supplement manufacturing process, or even during transit to a retail store, can result in a product with practically no living probiotics on the store shelf. This is why it is so important to select supplemental probiotic products from a manufacturer you can trust. Probiotic supplements made to higher quality standards tend to survive longer and through more adverse conditions than poor quality probiotic supplements. So stick with brands you can trust.

Lifestyle

Increasing nutritional intake and dabbling in herbal medicine are great ways to start building up our natural defenses, but any immune-bolstering program should also include overall healthy lifestyle changes.

Exercise

Getting a minimum of 30 minutes of exercise four to five days a week is a realistic goal to help activate the immune system in a number of different ways, including enhancing T-cell and antibody responses and boosting circulation so defender cells get where they need to go. Exercise also helps to reduce emotional stress by regulating the stress hormone cortisol, which is believed to weaken the immune system.

Stress Reduction

Stress is the immune system's natural enemy, flooding the body with neurochemicals that make white blood cells sluggish and weak. In addition to exercise, try engaging in activities like yoga, tai chi, guided imagery, and healthy time-management in order to foster relaxation and spiritual balance.

Ditch the Vices

Excessive alcohol, sugar, and smoking have all been associated with diminished immune system performance.

Improve Your Diet

Loading up on nutrient-dense whole foods, especially antioxidant-rich colorful fruits and vegetables, can deliver immune-boosting nutrition and inflammation-modulating compounds.

Get Enough Rest

The number one health recommendation. Inadequate sleep weakens immune performance; getting enough sleep helps to modulate and balance the immune system, enabling it to recharge and function properly.

Wash Your Hands

Common sense steps should not be overlooked, especially when it comes to cold and flu season. Avoid contagious people, wash hands frequently, and even use a handkerchief on common surfaces like doorknobs and shopping cart handles. By sidestepping pathogens, you can give your immune system a break and enable your healing energies to recharge.

THE FOUR HALLMARKS OF QUALITY BOTANICAL SUPPLEMENTS

One of the ways you can improve your results from taking the immune-boosting botanical medicines recommended in this book is to ensure that the herbal supplements you buy are of the highest quality possible. But how can you tell? For example, most people don't have an analytical laboratory at their disposal where they can check the quality of a dietary supplement. Even if they did, most wouldn't have a clue how to use it. And, since a supplement's immune-boosting effects are not necessarily a property you can feel, how can your average non-scientists know that they're getting a top quality supplement? In fact, there are four hallmarks of quality that botanical supplement shoppers should look for. These are:

- Standardization
- Inclusion of whole herb (whole active plant part)
- Proper delivery
- Independent laboratory testing

Many botanical supplement brands get high marks on one or two of these hallmarks. But only the best can claim all four. So, for peak immune-boosting performance, look for a brand that covers all four of these hallmarks of quality.

Standardization

Once a novel concept in the botanical supplements

market, standardization is the future. It enables supplement manufacturers to provide a quality product that consumers can trust. Standardization is the identification and quantification of an active or biochemical marker compound, which assures the product is of the correct quality. These extracts are many times more concentrated than the raw herb. Also, in many cases, the process of standardization and increasing the concentration of active principles tends to eliminate contaminants such as pesticides. But standardization is just the first step in the guarantee of efficacy because, even with standardization:

- A product may not be bioavailable enough to be adequately absorbed.
- The product could be standardized to a lesser percentage of chemical marker compound or not have enough of the ingredient in the bottle.

That is why it is so important that you use products you can trust from manufacturers who are buying the best raw materials and manufacturing them correctly into the desired final product.

Thirty years ago, when you could only find botanical supplements at your local health food store, most of these supplements gave no indication of the identity or quantity of an herb's active constituents. For example, a bottle of ginseng capsules would simply indicate that each capsule contained some milligram amount of ginseng. Better-quality botanical supplements sometimes indicated the plant part used, for example, that each capsule contained, say, 400 mg of ginseng root. But few gave any further information.

The only valid method of describing the potency of an herb is to identify at least one bioactive constituent or activity marker of that herb and report its concentration. Ginseng, for example, contains ginsenosides. And studies have shown that a sample of ginseng root with twice the ginsenosides of another has twice the energizing activity of that other ginseng root. Likewise, a sample with four times the ginsenosides has four times the activity. In this case, ginsenosides are known to be active constituents, and comparing various ginseng supplements by the milligram quantity of ginsenosides gives a reasonable estimation of the relative potency. So a supplement with 12.5 mg of ginsenosides per serving will likely deliver twice the energizing activity of one that delivers only 6.25 mg of ginsenosides.

I mentioned the term "activity marker" as an alternative constituent of an herb which can be used as a measure of true activity. An activity marker constituent is used when science has not yet identified a compound or group of compounds responsible for an herb's activity. St. John's Wort, for example, contains hypericin, which is responsible for some, but not all, of the herb's antidepressant effects. Other St. John's Wort constituents, such as hyperforin, have been found to display significant activity. Exactly which compound or group of compounds is most responsible for the herb's effects is still unknown. But what is known is that if your sample of St. John's Wort extract naturally contains more hypericin, then it will naturally contain high concentrations of the other active constituents, and the empirical evidence shows it will have a higher potency that is proportional with such hypericin concentration. Thus hypericin can be viewed as a marker constituent.

The phenomenon behind the fact that marker constituent concentrations can reliably determine relative potency is very basic to key ideals of good standardization. A properly standardized herbal extract is one in which the herb has been grown under optimal conditions, harvested at peak potency, and extracted using simple laboratory methods of concentration and purification. Farmers are always under pressure to plant more herbs per acre in order to maximize profitability. Likewise, they are under pressure to minimize costly irrigation, neglect soil nutrient status, and not go to the expense of growing healthy herbs. It's the same in any type of farming. With fruits and vegetables, we can taste the inferior quality of produce such practices yield. If we want poor quality fruits and vegetables, we know where to buy them and how much they cost. If we want good quality produce, we know where to buy them as well. But with herbal extracts sold in capsules, it's more difficult because you can't taste the quality. Standardization gives a us a good clue.

With many herbs, it is not cost effective to try to achieve higher milligram concentrations of active constituents from poorly grown herbs. If you are trying to achieve 20% oleuropein in a finished olive leaf extract, you have to perform a lot less work by starting out with olive leaves that contain 6% oleuropein than by starting out with 3% leaves. But take care that you are not buying a product where just one constituent is apparently higher, because some manufacturers will spike the active constituent chemical from other sources. If you demand standardization together with the other hallmarks of quality described in this chapter, you won't go wrong. For example, as I explain in the next section, it's important to have the whole active part of the herb.

Whole Herb

Inclusion of whole herb (or the active part of the plant, such as whole leaf) is an important factor in determining the quality of an herbal extract. As I alluded to earlier in this chapter, science often does not know all of the active constituents in a therapeutic herb. Usually, there is not only a primary active constituent but also a number of important cofactors that help that constituent do its job. Including whole herb is the only way to ensure that all of the unknown active cofactors are included in the herbal extract.

The concept is best illustrated by the discovery of bioflavonoids. Prior to the 20th Century, vitamin C was unknown, and seafarers achieved the now-recognized vitamin C effects (preventing or curing scurvy) by eating limes and other citrus fruits while at sea. Hence, British sailors were called limeys. Along with the 20th Century came the notion that more is better. And to make a long story short, a Hungarian researcher and clinician named Albert Szent-Györgyi had the notion that 100% pure vitamin C would cure scurvy better and faster than 90% pure vitamin C from citrus fruit. He discovered that this notion was wrong. It was found that 90% pure vitamin C contains other, as yet unknown, citrus cofactors, which vastly improved vitamin C's anti-scorbutic (scurvy-curing) activity. Without those cofactors, the pure vitamin C hardly worked as expected. These cofactors were later identified as bioflavonoids, and they illustrated how important it is to include whole fruit, or herb as the case may be, in your therapeutic botanical supplements. The truth is that our science is very young, and we have yet to identify, much less understand, all of the important cofactors that belong in a therapeutic herbal supplement. So keeping the complete botanical medicine signature of the plant in the supplement ensures that none are lost.

Proper Delivery:
Extended Release vs. Rapid Release

With botanical supplementation, it will often suffice

to administer an extract in common capsule or tablet form. But in many cases, particularly when you are trying to achieve maximum benefit, it is better to extend the release of that extract to achieve longer lasting benefits and/or greater absorption of active principles. For maximum immune-boosting benefits, you should consider taking olive leaf extract, ARA-Larix, and *Andrographis paniculata* extract in extended release delivery form.

It used to be nearly impossible to find botanical supplements in any delivery system aside from the common, rapid-release forms: capsules, tablets, soft-gels, liquids, teas, and tinctures. But in the 1980s, it was discovered that natural vegetable cellulose could be employed to prolong the release of medicines or botanical supplements. In so doing, the medicine or herb could be released from a tablet over the course of 8 to 12 hours, depending on the concentration of cellulose. This could be useful for therapeutic agents that were required to perform for many hours at a time. This extended delivery method was also found to have another valuable property, which was to increase the amount of the therapeutic agent absorbed into the bloodstream from the gastrointesti-nal tract. In some cases, the absorption of the thera-peutic agent was found to increase by 40% over that of regular rapid-release tablets and capsules. Vitamin C is just such an example.

Using natural vegetable cellulose to prolong the release of nutrients is not a new phenomenon. In fact, it is the way Mother Nature has done it for millions of years. When we eat foods, our teeth and stomach break large pieces of food into smaller chunks. But the smaller chunks are actually enormous on the molecular scale. The nutrients in a piece of carrot just a few hundredths of a millimeter across come as nutrient molecules (beta carotene for example) embedded within a matrix or meshwork of plant fiber. It takes many hours for our digestive systems to liberate the nutrients from the natural vegetable cellulose matrix of the fragment of carrot. Naturally, our digestive system is perfectly suited to absorb nutrients released slowly from such food matrices.

Only recently have we begun to put medicines and nutrients into capsules and tablets. Common tablets and capsules add convenience, but in some instances, immediate release of all the active ingredients may not be desired. Being able to release a nutrient into the intestine to be absorbed over time can help with overall delivery into the bloodstream.

Extending the release of nutrients has not been tested on most herbs for validation that it actually improves absorption. However, it has been tested on a number of drugs and nutrients such as vitamin C, and has been found to bestow 40% greater absorption into the bloodstream. So, because prolonging release confers a more natural dispersion within the intestines and may enhance bioavailability, it is a nice feature to have in a supplement.

But, even without 40% greater absorption, there are other good reasons to go with an extended release supplement, if available. Not only is extended release likely to improve absorption, but because it spreads the nutrient release out over many hours, it is also likely to be gentler on the gastrointestinal tract. Extended release reduces the likelihood that any single area of the GI tract will have an extremely high concentration of any particular nutrient.

With these key benefits (prolonged therapeutic activity and increased absorption), a few top-quality supplement manufacturers adopted the technology and began to offer supplements in extended delivery form.

Independent Laboratory Testing

I cannot stress enough the importance of choosing a supplement with independent verification of quality. As I alluded to earlier in this chapter, some hallmarks of quality may be misrepresented and misunderstood. For example, standardization may give the appearance of superiority to a botanical supplement, simply by playing up the illusion that more is better. So I never recommend relying on the printed standardization alone. I like to see inclusion of whole herb/active plant part printed on the label as well. But the most important hallmark of quality that I look for in addition to standardization is independent laboratory verification of quality.

I want to know that qualified chemical analysts, other than those employed by the manufacturer, have tested the supplement and given it the thumbs up. While there may be many botanical supplement manufacturers willing to take liberties with exaggerations and misrepresentations on their labels, it would be very difficult for such companies to get an independent laboratory, with its own reputation on the line, to validate such deceptions as well. An independent laboratory's certificate of analysis is truly of inestimable value.

Just how widespread is the problem of inaccurate labels? It's so bad that the cheaters have government regulations on their side. The U.S. Code of Federal Regulations 21CFR101.36 (f), 101.9 (g) revision of April 2008, actually allows manufacturers to put in 20% less of any ingredient(s) than their label claims.

If that weren't bad enough, careless supplement manufacturers can further diminish the potency of a product—by 60% or more—by including impurities or permitting excess moisture during production, improper storage conditions throughout the manufacturing process, and improper packaging. And if you think that carelessness is just a habit of the unsuccessful, think again. Being careless costs a company less than being careful does. I have interviewed supplement manufacturers and have heard the stories of the good, the bad, and the ugly. When it comes to supplement manufacturing, careless is definitely less costly than careful. There's less cleaning; but a quality manufacturer must ensure that its manufacturing machinery is thoroughly cleaned before and after making every batch of every product. There's less double-checking; but a quality manufacturer never takes for granted that an ingredient meets all of its specifications: It double checks, analyzes, tests, and retests. There's less quality assurance; but a quality manufacturer employs a staff of quality assurance technicians who not only perform the testing, but check to make sure that everyone else in the production process is checking and double-checking properly. With careless manufacturing, there are no shelf-life and stability considerations; but a quality manufacturer performs accelerated shelf-life testing and real-time shelf-life testing on its products so that customers can be sure that the product they've purchased is good even three years after it was produced. Careless manufacturing saves money for the manufacturer, but it is the consumer who suffers, sometimes getting less than half of the potency they paid for. I am a firm believer in opting for an established brand I can trust, one that meets all of the hallmarks of quality I've described.

CONCLUSION

The natural health revolution is underway. Of all the myriad modalities, herbs, nutrients, and lifestyle changes in the natural health sphere, one unifying philosophy prevails: Preventing illness is far preferable to treating illness. While modern science has made tremendous leaps and bounds forward in terms of treating illness, it has reached a dead end in a number of conditions—everything from the common cold to incurable diseases.

And with that, humanity has come full circle in terms of health. Rather than seeking solutions in laboratory-born synthetic substances, many are turning inward, seeking to strengthen and optimize the defense that nature gave us: the immune system. The ultimate preventive health tool, this complex network has practiced, refined, and adapted over the course of millions of years—all in order to fulfill its noble mission of protecting you against the millions of bacteria, viruses, and parasites that assault your body every day.

Unfortunately, in the eternal battle of immunity versus pathogens, the modern world has given a distinct advantage to the bad guys. As humankind has separated itself from its true natural state, the immune system's delicate balance has been thrown off-kilter. Bombarded by environmental toxins, crippled by stress, starved of nutrition, and weakened by reliance on synthetic drugs, the immune system malfunctions. As a result, the immune system either underperforms, leaving the body susceptible to invading pathogens, or overreacts and attacks the body's own cells, leading to autoimmune disease.

It's a distressing revelation: We may be at a point in history where the very world that we have created is crippling our primary defense against sickness. While these immune-damaging factors escalate, super bugs evolve and mutate—painting a bleak health scenario for both the present day and the future.

However, we have the power to lend a helping hand to the immune system that works so tirelessly to protect us. As is so often the case, nature provides antidotes that are far more sophisticated than what our most advanced laboratories can create. Throughout this book we've discussed three such natural marvels. Olive leaf, ARA-Larix, and *Andrographis paniculata* are natural botanicals, actually gifts from nature with a remarkable capacity to stimulate the immune system, modulate the immune response, and promote health across numerous other body systems. As remarkable as these immune-boosting herbs are on their own, they work even better when used together. But for the greatest immune support of all, consider a lifestyle approach that incorporates the healthy shifts in habits suggested in Chapter 9.

As the natural health philosophy advances and preventive health moves to the fore, immune function takes center stage. For many, immune function has always meant one thing: Overcoming the common cold or influenza. But the emergence of super bugs, mysterious pandemic super-flu scenarios, and ever-present threat of chronic disease have elevated proper immune function to a whole new level of significance. More than ever, our immunity represents our salvation from all that ails us—from minor infections to life-threatening illnesses.

Our modern achievements, however, have created a world that disables our immune systems—leaving our defenses down against both known and unknown pathogen threats. That's where natural immune-builders like olive leaf, ARA-Larix, and andrographis come in. Along with abundant nutrition and healthy lifestyle changes, olive leaf, ARA-Larix, and andrographis represent a way to balance out the environmental assaults on our immune systems. With these remarkable botanicals, we can neutralize harmful toxins and microbes, replacing them instead with safe, natural nutrition that boosts immunity, gently modulates immunity, and otherwise supports numerous immune system functions. For all the immune system does to protect us and support our well-being, the least we can do is repay it in kind—and olive leaf, ARA-Larix, and andrographis are the perfect way to start.

ABOUT THE AUTHOR

Dr. Jim LaValle is an educator, clinician, and consultant in the field of integrative health care. Dr. LaValle is a licensed pharmacist (University of Cincinnati College of Pharmacy), board certified clinical nutritionist (International & American Associations of Clinical Nutritionists, [IAACN]), and doctor of naturopathic medicine (Central States College of Health Sciences), with more than twenty years clinical practice experience in the field of natural therapeutics and functional medicine.

Dr. LaValle was named one of the "50 Most Influential Druggists" by *American Druggist* for his work in natural medicine in 1998. Dr. LaValle is the founder of LaValle Metabolic Institute, Cincinnati, OH, and a nationally-recognized speaker and media personality. His experience ranges from extensive clinical practice, product design and formulation, and technology development, to author, educator, and media personality.

Dr. LaValle is currently Adjunct Associate Professor at the University of Cincinnati College of Pharmacy. He has developed educational programs for Rite Aid, McKesson, and Longs Drugs, among others, and trains independent pharmacists and physicians about natural medicine. He is a past contributor to *Drug Store News* and *Retail Pharmacy News*, in addition to radio and television programming.

He has also authored 12 other books, including *Smart Medicine for Healthier Living, Drug-Induced Nutrient Depletion Handbook* and *The Cholestin Breakthrough,* and co-authored *The Nutritional Cost of Prescription Drugs* and *Natural Therapeutics Pocket Guide.*

INDEX

124 *Botanicals for Immunity*